TEXTBOOK OF PHYSIOLOGY
FOR HOMOEOPATHIC STUDENTS

TEXTBOOK OF PHYSIOLOGY

FOR HOMOEOPATHIC STUDENTS

Dr. Harbakhash Singh Sandhar
*Dean, Canadian College of Homoeopathic Medicine,
Alberta, Canada*

CONTRIBUTORS

- Brijinder Singh, MD
- Rohit Jain, BHMS
- Nitin Shakya, MBBS
- Taru Bhagat, BHMS
- Anil Kumar Kandpal, MBBS

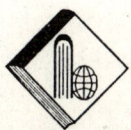

B. JAIN PUBLISHERS PVT. LTD.

TEXTBOOK OF PHYSIOLOGY
(FOR HOMOEOPATHIC STUDENTS)

First Edition : 2004

All rights are reserved. No part of this book may be reproduced, stored in a retrieval system or transmitted, in any form or by any means, mechanical, photocopying, recording or otherwise, without any prior written permission of the publishers.

© Copyright with the Publishers

Price: Rs. 225.00

Published by Kuldeep Jain for
B. Jain Publishers (P) Ltd.
1921, Street No. 10, Chuna Mandi,
Paharganj, New Delhi - 110 055 (INDIA)
Phones: 2358 0800, 5169 8991, 2358 3100, 2358 1300, 2358 1100
Fax: 2358 0471, 5169 8993; *Email:* bjain@vsnl.com
Website: www.bjainbooks.com

Printed in India by
J.J. Offset Printers
522, FIE, Patpar Ganj, Delhi - 110 092
Phones: 22169633, 22156128

ISBN : 81-8056-414-2

BOOK CODE : BS-5746

PREFACE

Textbook of Physiology (For Homoeopathic Students) is my third contribution in the series of books which I have planned for homoeopathic students. Like my earlier two books, viz. *Textbook of Orthalmology and Otology* and *Textbook of Pathology, Bacteriology and Parasitology*, this book is meant for BHMS students and is strictly according the Central Council of Homoeopathy (CCH) Syllabus.

The book has been written and designed to introduce the students to the basic concepts of physiology.

There are many good books on physiology written by experienced authors but they are too bulky and the language is also difficult for homoeopathy undergraduates.

This book covers all the topics as per CCH syllabus in a synstematic manner. Moreover, it is full of *diagrams* and *flow charts*, which are essential for the students to understand the subject better.

I have prefusely consulted all the major physiology books presently in the market in the making of this book. Thus ensuring that no important concept gets missed out.

At the end of the book important questions – both for *written exam ination* as well as *viva* are given. Also, I have provided some Multiple Choice Questions.

There are two Appendices — Appendix-I contains investigations with normal values and Appendix-II contains some commonly used abbreviations.

I hope this book will help the readers during their student as well as clinical life.

Dr. Harbakhash Singh Sandhar
Dean, Canadian College of Homoeopathic Medicine,
Alberta, Canada

BOOKS CONSULTED IN THE MAKING OF THIS BOOK

1. *Principles of Anatomy and Physiology* by Tortora and Grabowski.
2. *Human Physiology (The basis of Medicine)* by Gillian Pockock.
3. *Human Physiology (The mechanisms of body function)* by Vanden, Sherman and Luciano.
4. *Human Physiology* by C.C. Chatterjee.
5. *Review of Medical Physiology* by William F. Ganong – 19th edition.
6. *Textbook of Physiology* by Prof. A.K. Jain.
7. *Textbook of Human Physiology* by Guyton.
8. Internet Resources.

CONTENTS

Preface 03

Books consulted 04

Introduction to physiology 11-13

Chapter-1 : TRANSPORT MECHANISMS ....(15-18)
- Introduction 15
- Active transport process 15
- Passive transport process 17

Chapter-2 : BODY TISSUES ....(19-28)
- Introduction 19
- Epithilial tissues 19
- Connective tissues 20
- Muscle tissues 20
- Nervous tissues 28

Chapter-3 : BIO-CHEMICAL AND BIO-PHYSICAL PRINCIPLES ....(29-44)
- Matter 29
- Ions 29
- Isotopes 29
- Molecules 30
- Radicle 30
- Compounds 30
- Salts 30
- Electrolytes 30
- Osmosis 30
- Diffusion 31
- Filtration 32
- Cells 32
- Mitosis 35
- Meiosis 38
- Cancer 40
- Measuring concentrations of solution 40

- Ions 41
- Electrolytes 41
- Non-electrolytes 41
- Filteration 42
- Absorption 42
- Donan equilibrium 42
- Acids 42
- Colloids 43
- Surface tensions 43
- Bases 43
- Enzymes 43

Chapter-4 : PROTEINS, CARBOHYDRATES AND LIPIDS ....(45-50)
- Proteins 45
- Carbohydrates 46
- Lipids 47

Chapter-5 : NUTRITION AND HEALTH ....(51-58)
- Introduction 51
- Classification of food 51
- Nutrients 52
- Proteins 52
- Fats 53
- Carbohydrate 53
- Vitamins 54

Chapter-6 : THE BLOOD ....(59-77)
- Introduction 59
- Composition 59
- Blood cells 60
- Anaemias 62
- White blood cells of W.B.C. or leucocytes 63
- Platelets 65
- Summary of formed elements in blood 66
- Haemostasis 66
- Blood volume 70
- R.B.C. indices 71
- Plasma proteins 72
- Haemoglobin 73
- Blood group 74
- Jaundice 75

Chapter-7	:	THE RETICULOENDOTHELIAL SYSTEM ....(79-82)

- Recticuloendothelial of circulation 80
- Lymph 80
- Spleen 81
- Lymph nodes 81
- Edema 82

Chapter-8	:	THE CARDIOVASCULAR SYSTEM ....(83-111)

- Organisation of circulation 84
- Functions of circulation 84
- Cardiac muscle 85
- Cardiac cycle 85
- Heart sound 87
- What is apex beat 88
- ECG 89
- Blood distribution at rest 91
- Cardiac output 92
- Haemodynamics 96
- Pecullarites of cerebral circulation 99
- Pulmonary circulation 100
- Skin circulation 101
- Triple response 101
- Cardiovascular regulation 102
- Baroreceptors 104
- Chemoreceptors 105
- Shock 106
- Cardiac impulse 107
- The vascular system 109
- Blood flow 110
- Cushing reaction 111
- Cardiac depression 111

Chapter-9	:	THE DIGESTIVE SYSTEM ....(113-136)

- Introduction 114
- Metabolism 114
- Human breast milk 115
- Digestive system 116
- Gastrointestinal tract 117
- Functions of oral cavity 119
- Stomach 121
- Vomiting 125
- Small intestine 125
- Large intestine 128

- Liver 129
- Diet 131
- Digestion and absorption in the git 132
- Absorption of fluids / electrolytes / vitamins 135
- Biological value (B.V.) 136

Chapter-10 : THE INTEGUMENTARY SYSTEM ....(137-141)
- Introduction 137
- The skin 138
- Glands 138
- Body temperature regulation 140

Chapter-11 : THE RESPIRATORY SYSTEM ....(142-164)
- Introduction 143
- Anatomy 144
- Nervous control 145
- Local factors 145
- Respiratory membrane 145
- Nose 146
- Pleura 146
- The respiratory unit 147
- Respiratory movements 147
- Alveolar pressure 148
- Pulmonary volumes 149
- Dynamic pulmonary volume 149
- Spirometry 150
- Compliance of the lungs 150
- Surfactant 151
- Vocalization 151
- Cough reflex 153
- Respiratory quotient 153
- Composition of inspired and expired air 153
- Respiration control 154
- Transport of oxygen and carbon dioxide 155
- Gas exchange between blood and tissues 159
- Apnoea 160
- Cheyne-strokes respiration 160
- Dyspnoea 161
- Cyanosis 161
- Asphyxia 161
- Acclimatization 162
- Artifical respiration 163
- Caisson's disease 163

Chapter-12 :	THE EXCRETORY SYSTEM ....(165-178)	

- Kidneys 166
- Micturition 166
- Mechanism of formation of urine 166
- Physiological anatomy of the kidneys....................................166
- Blood flow to the kidney 168
- Urine formation 169
- Micturition reflex 170
- Renal functions 170
- Juxta transport mechanism 170
- Clearance 172
- Renal transport mechanism 172
- Diuretics 176
- Kidney function tests 176

Chapter-13 :	THE NERVOUS SYSTEM ....(179-208)	

- Introduction 180
- Peripheral nervous system 181
- Action potential propagation 183
- Synapse 184
- Neuro transmitters 185
- Receptors 185
- Reflex 185
- Sensory pathways 187
- Motor pathway 189
- Autonomic nervous system 192
- Body posture 194
- Vestibular system 198
- Reticular formation 198
- Limbic system 199
- Basal ganglia 199
- Hydrothalamus 201
- Electro encephalogram 202
- Sleep 203
- Cerebellium 205
- Cerebrospinal fluid system 206
- Conditional reflexes 207
- Circadian rhythm 207
- Speech 208
- Learning 208
- Some important terms 208

Chapter-14 : THE SENSE ORGANS ....(209-229)
- The eye 210
- Taste 221
- Smell 223
- Ear 224
- The larynx 227

Chapter-15 : ENDOCRINE SYSTEM ....(231-246)
- Introduction 232
- Differences between endocrine system and nervous system 232
- Hormones 232
- Hypothalamus 234
- Pituritary glands 235
- Thyroid glands 237
- Adenal glands 240
- Islets of langerhans 244
- Aging and the endocrine system 246

Chapter-16 : REPRODUCTION ....(247-261)
- Introduction 247
- Male reproductive system 247
- Female reproductive system 251
- The breast 257
- Embryogenesis 260
- Homologus structures of the male and female reproductive system 261

Important questions 263-266

Multiple choice question 267-274

Appendix I & II 275-277

List of figures 278-282

INDRODUCTION TO PHYSIOLOGY

PHYSIOLOGY

It is the science that deals with the functions of living organism and its parts. It is a combination of two Greek words (Physis which means "nature" and logos which means "science").

CHARACTERISTICS OF LIFE

Life is defined by a list of attributes that taken together are known as characteristic of life.

These characteristic are :

1. Responsiveness
2. Conductivity
3. Respiration
4. Digestion and absorption
5. Secretion and excretion
6. Growth
7. Reproduction

LEVEL OF ORGANISATION

Overview

Human physiology is concerned with correct functioning of various organ systems. Organs are finally made up of cells. The cells are, therefore, the basic unit of life. It is the smallest unit capable of an independent existence. The study of cells is known as cytology.

Most cells are microscopic and their size ranges from 10-30 micrometers. Cells have five principle components :

1. Plasma membrane
2. Cytoplasm
3. Nucleus
4. Organelles
5. Inclusions

The human body is orgnaised at different levels. The simpler level is followed by a functionally and structurally more complex higher level.

Man
Make up ↑↓ Composed of
Organ System
E.g. Respiratory system

↑↓

Organs, e.g. Lungs

↑↓

Tissues
E.g. Epithelial tissue

↑↓

Cells, e.g. Squamous cells, columuar cells, etc.

↑↓

Organelles
E.g. Endoplasmic reticulum

↑↓

Macromolecules
E.g. lipoproteins

↑↓

Small molecules, e.g. fatty acids

↑↓

Atoms of the element

HOMEOSTASIS

In 1932, a famous American physiologist, Walter B. Cannon, suggested the name "homeostasis" for a relatively constant state maintained by the body. The word has two Greek words (Homoios which means "The same" and stasis which means "standing").

Homeostasis maintenance means that the cells of the body are in an environment that meets their needs and permit them to function normally under changing external conditions. The mechanism or device which maintains or restores homeostasis is known as homeostatic control mechanism. To accomplish this self-regulation, a highly complex and integrated communication control system or network is required and this is called as the *feedback control loop*.

There are a minimum of three basic components in every feedback control loop:

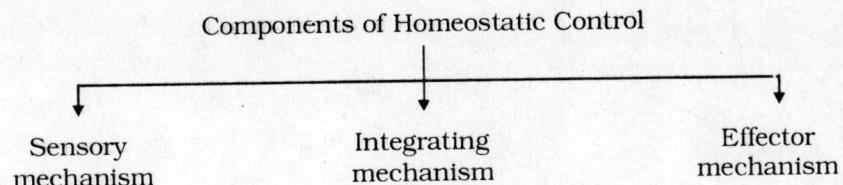

Interactions between the various body systems (Respiratory, Cardiovascular, Lymphatic, Nervous, Digestive, Urinary, Reproductive, Skeletal, Endocrine) contribute to the homeostasis of the body as a whole.

EDUCATION, EXPERIENCE AND MEMORIES ARE THREE THINGS NO ONE CAN TAKE AWAY FROM YOU.

1
TRANSPORT MECHANISMS

INTRODUCTION

In order to survive, a cell must be able to transport its substances from within outwards and from outside to inside. The membrane transport processes can be divided as :

I. Active
II. Passive

ACTIVE TRANSPORT PROCESS

They require expenditure of energy for transportation.

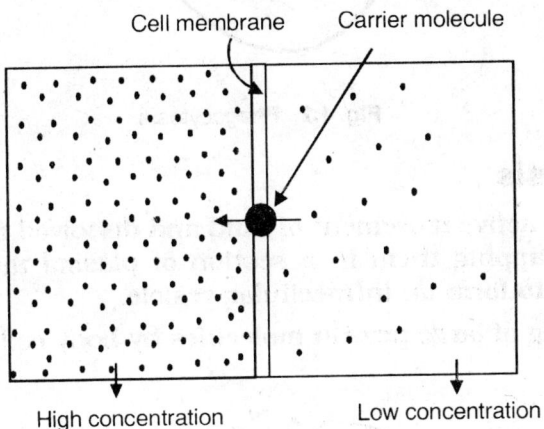

Fig. 1.1 Active process.

It is movement of solute particles from an area of low concentration to an area of high concentration, i.e., against the concentration gradient by means of a carrier.

E.g. Na^+ / K^+ ATPase Pump

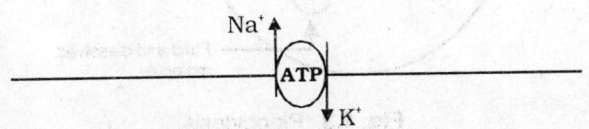

Na$^+$/K$^+$ ATPase pump breaks down the ATP Molecules to ADP molecules and the energy released by this process is used for active transport of ions across the cell-membrane. Coupling ratio of this pump is 3 : 2 which means that for each molecule of ATP that is broken 3 Na$^+$ move out of the cell and 2 K$^+$ enter the cell.

Phagocytosis

It is an active process of movement of cells or other large particles into cell by trapping it in a section of plasma membrane that pinches off to form an intracellular vesicle.

E.g. W.B.C. trap the bacterial cells by the mechanism of phagocytosis.

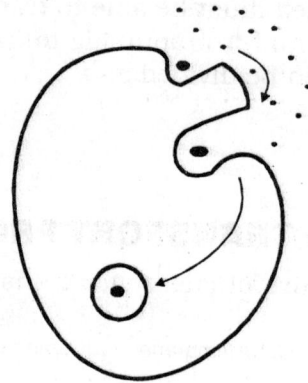

Fig. 1.2 Phagocytosis.

Pinocytosis

It is also an active movement of fluid and dissolved molecules into a cell by trapping them in a section of plasma membrane that pinches off to form an intracellular vesicle.

E.g. trapping of large protein molecules by body cells.

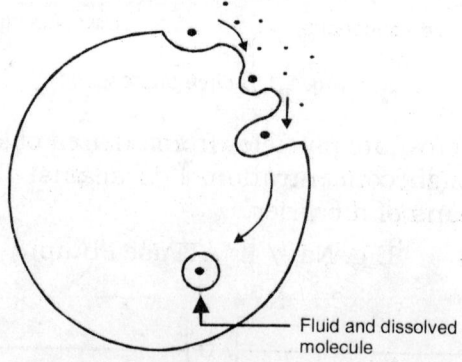

Fig. 1.3 Pinocytosis.

Exocytosis

It is an active transport mechanism of movement of products out of the cells by fusing a secretory vesicle with the plasma membrane.

E.g. secretion of certain proteins, hormones etc.

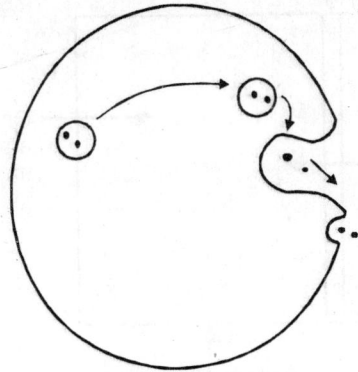

Fig. 1.4 Exocytosis.

PASSIVE TRANSPORT PROCESS

It does not require any energy. The movement of particles occurs along the concentration gradient, i.e. from higher to lower concentration.

Diffusion

Movement of particles through the phospholipid bilayer or through channels from an area of high concentration to an area of low concentration, e.g., CO_2 movement out of all the cells.

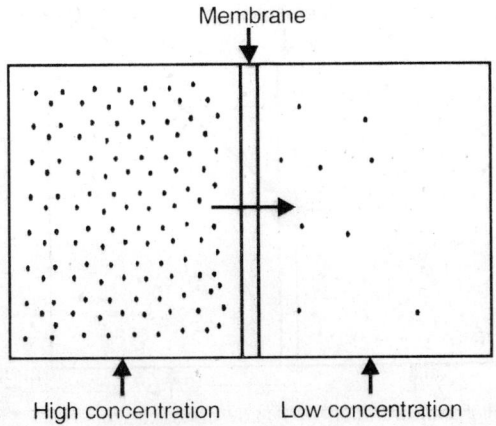

Fig. 1.5 Diffusion.

Dialysis

It is diffusion of small solute particles, through a selectively permeable membrane.

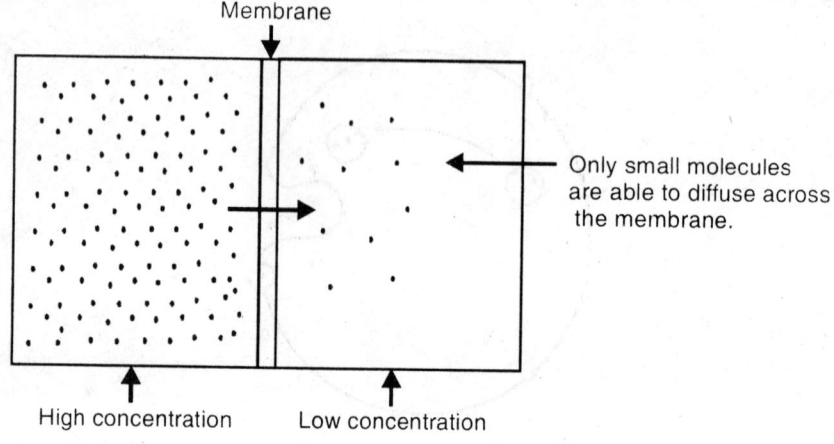

Fig. 1.6 Dialysis.

Osmosis

It is the movement of water from a region of low solute concentration or in other words it is movement of water from a region of high water concentration to a region of low water concentration.

Facilitated diffusion

It uses a carrier molecule, therefore, this process is also known as carrier-mediated passive transport. E.g. facilitated transport for glucose.

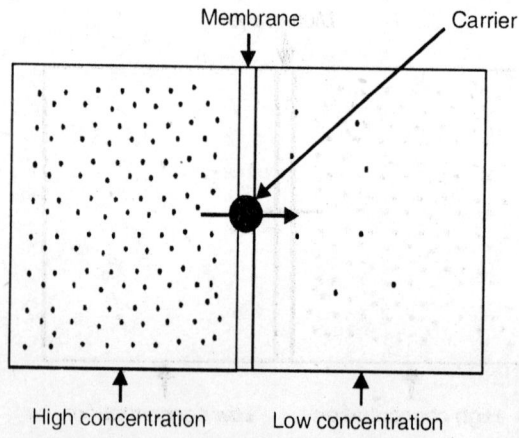

Fig. 1.7 Facilitated diffusion.

2

BODY TISSUES

INTRODUCTION

A tissue is a group of similar cells that perform a common function.

Origin of tissues

All tissues of the body are derived from 3 primary germ layers – Endoderm, Ectoderm and Mesoderm.

Types

1. Epithilial tissue
2. Connective tissue
3. Muscle tissue
4. Nervous tissue

EPITHELIAL TISSUES
[All the 3 germ layers contribute to epithelical tissue]

Epithilial tissue (epithelium) consists of cells arranged in sheets either single or multilayered. Cells of the epithelium rest on a layer of extracellular matrix, called the basement membrane. Epithelial tissue is avascular and exchange of substances between it and the comective tissue occurs by diffusion across the basement membrane. Epithelal tissue has a nerve supply.

Types

1. Covering and lining epithelium.
2. Glandular epithelium.

Functions

1. Protection
2. Secretion
3. Absorption
4. Excretion

5. Filtration
6. Gaseous exchange (in lungs)

In ear, nose and eye certain epithelial structures are specialised to act as sensory structures, for hearing, smell and vision respectively.

CONNECTIVE TISSUES
[Derived from Mesoderm]

It is the most widespread tissues in the body, found in or around nearly every organ of the body.

Types

1. Fibrous
2. Bone
3. Cartilage
4. Blood

Functions

1. It connects together, supports and strengthens the other internal organs.
2. Protects the various internal organs.
3. Compartmentalizes structures such as skeletal muscles.
4. Transports the various substances to and from various body parts (blood, fluid).
5. Providing immunity to body.

MUSCLE TISSUE
[Derived from mesoderm, mostly]

Types

1. Skeletal muscle
2. Smooth muscle
3. Cardiac muscle

Functions

1. Producing body movements.
2. Maintaining the body posture.
3. Urine is stored in urinary bladder; similarly food is stored in stomach temporarily for digestion. This storage is possible due to sphincteric action of muscle fibers located at their outlet.

4. Contraction of smooth muscle fibers in the walls of intestines brings about the movement of food down the tract.
5. Contraction of cardiac muscle in the heart pumps the blood through the blood vessels.
6. Contraction of muscles in legs aid in return of blood to heart.

Properties

1. *Electrical excitability* — It is the ability of the muscle cells to produce action potentials in response to certain stimuli (electrial, chemical).
2. *Contractility* — It is the ability of muscle tissue to contract in response to an action potential. Muscle contraction can be either :
    (a) Isotonic muscle contraction (i.e. the tension developed remains constant while the muscle shortens).
    (b) Isometric muscle contraction (i.e. the tension developed increases while the length of muscle remains constant).
3. *Extensibility* — It is the ability of muscle to be stretched without being damaged.
4. *Elasticity* — It is the ability of muscle tissue to regain its original size and shape after contraction or extension.

Skeletal muscle

The fibrous sheath covering the whole muscle is called *Epimyesium*. Within the muscle, bundles of 10 to 100 muscle fibers are surrounded by fibrous sheath called *Perimyesium*. Similary each muscle fiber is surrouded by a thin sheath called the *Endomyesium*. Microscopic examination of a typical skeletal muscle reveals hundred and thousands of very long cylindrical cells called muscle fibers. These muscle fibres lie parallel to one another and range from 10 to 100 mm in diameter. The plasma membrane of a muscle cell is called *sarcolemma* and its surrounding cytoplasm is called *sarcoplasm*.

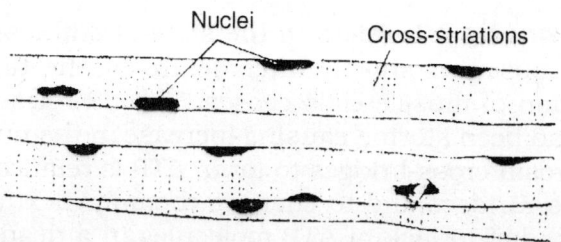

Fig. 2.1 Skeletal muscle

At high magnification the sarcoplasm appears stuffed with little threads. These small structures are the *myofibrils*. Although myofibrils extend lengthwise within the muscle fibre, their prominent alternative light and dark bands make the whole muscle fiber look striated or stripped. These bands are called cross striations.

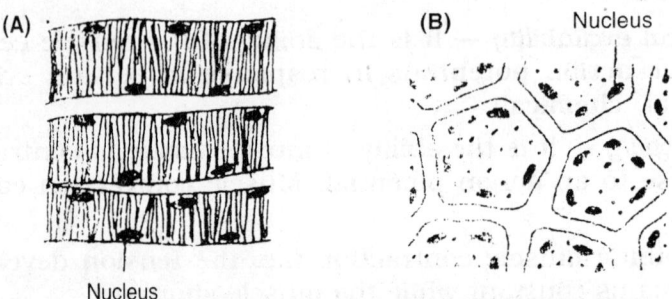

Fig. 2.2 A. Longitudinal section of skeletal muscle.
B. Transverse section of skeletal muscle.

Myofibrils which are the contractile elements of the skeletal muscle are 1-2 mm in diameter and contain three smaller structures called filaments. The thin filaments have 8 mm diameter as compared to thick filaments which have diameter of around 16 mm.

The filament do not extend the entire length of a muscle fiber. They are arranged in compartments called sarcomeres, which are the basic functional units of striated muscle fibres. Narrow plate-shaped region of dense material called Z line separates one sarcomere from the other. Within each sarcomere is A band which is darker and I band which is lighter. H zone in the centre of each A band contains thick but not thin filaments. M line divides the H zone.

The basic contractile proteins of the muscle are :

1. Actin
2. Myosin

Rigor mortis : It refers to the state of stiffness of skeletal muscles observed shortly after death. At the time of death stimulation of muscle cells ceases. The SR releases much of Ca^{2+} it had been storing causing increase in the number of the actin myosin cross-bridges to form. ATP is required to release the cross. Bridges and to energize them for next attachment. However, due to lack of ATP molecules in a dead body these cross-bridges are not released. Thus, due to the stuck bridges the dead body becomes stiffened.

How a skeletal muscle contracts

How a skeletal muscle contracts : The initial step is the stimulation of skeletal muscle by nerves. The nerve action potential causes release of acetylcholine which depolarise the muscle fiber membrane in the region adjacent to the end plate and this trigers muscle action potential which depolarizes T tubules and opens Ca^{2+} channels of sarcoplasmic reticulum and leads to increased sarcoplasmic Ca^{2+}. This in turn leads to skeletal muscle contraction. Now Ca^{2+} is pumped back into sarcoplasmic reticulum and this leads to muscle relaxation.

The process by which a muscle action potential triggers a contraction is known as *excitation – contraction coupling*.

Molecular events : The A band of each sarcomere consists mainly of myosin molecules arranged in thick

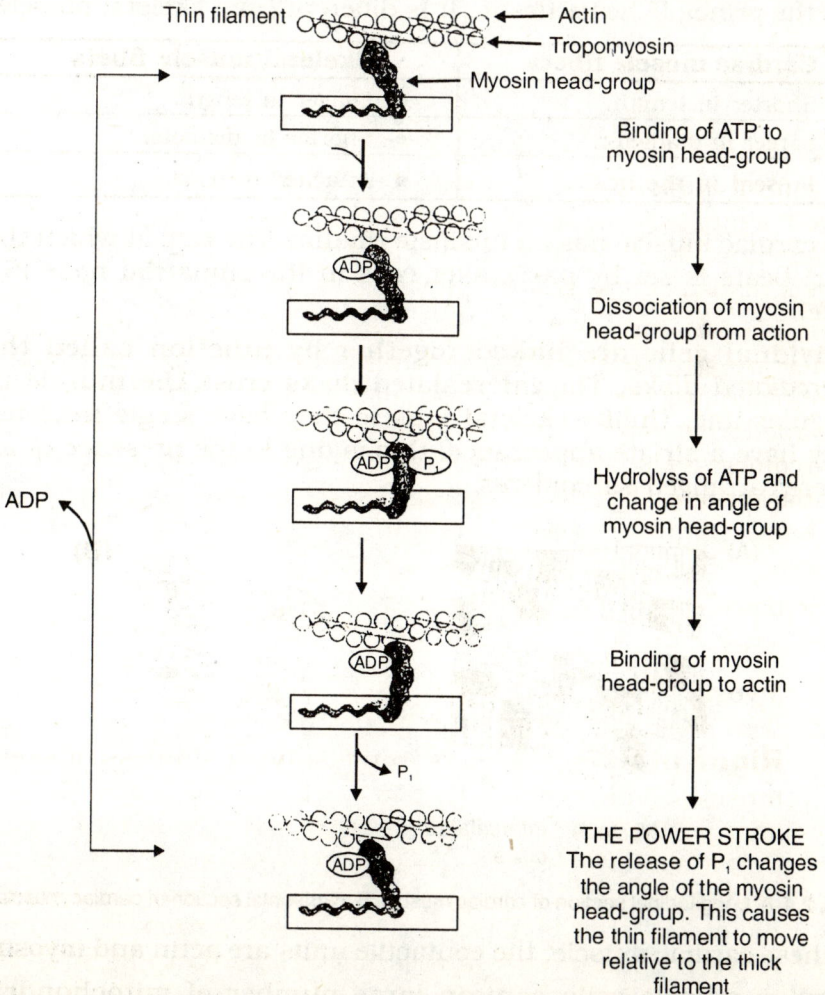

Fig. 2.3 Mechanism of muscle contraction.

filaments and I band consists mainly of actin, tropomyosin and troponin arranged in thin filament. The tension development occurs on interaction of actin and myosin. This can only occur when troponin complex binds calcium. This exposes the binding sites for myosin heads on actin.

When contraction occurs the actin and myosin form a series of cross-bridges that break and reform as ATP is hydrolyzed. As a result, the thick and thin filaments slide on each other and generation of force takes place.

This theory of muscle contraction is known as the *sliding filament theory* (given by Huxley and Huxley).

Cardiac muscle

It is the principle heart tissue. It is different from skeletal muscle.

Cardiac muscle fibers	Skeletal muscle fibers
• Shorter in length.	• Longer in length.
• Larger in diameter.	• Shorter in diameter.
• Present in the heart.	• Attached to bone.

The cardiac muscle has an intrinsic rhythm. The rate at which the heart beats is set by pacemaker cells in the sinuatrial node (SA node).

Individual cells are linked together by junction called the *intercalated disks*. The intercalated disks cross the muscle in irregular line. Unlike skeletal muscle they have single nucleus. They have a striate appearance; this is due to the presence of an orderly arranged sarcomeres.

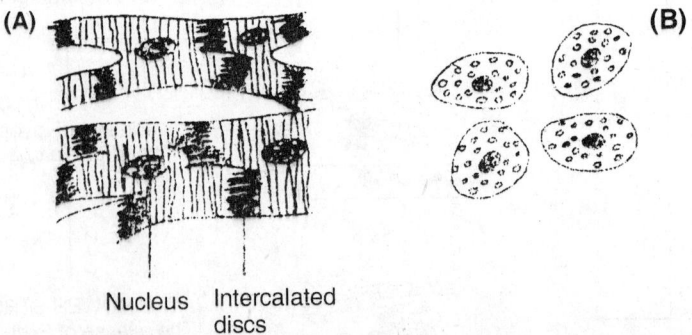

Fig. 2.4 A. Longitudinal section of cardiac muscle. B. Horizontal section of cardiac muscle.

In these cardiac muscle, the contactile units are actin and myosin.

Cardiac muscle cells contain large number of mitochondria distributed throughout the cytoplasm.

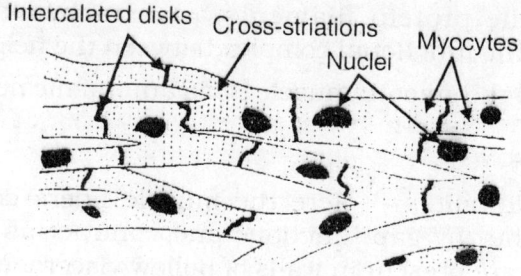

Fig. 2.5 Cardiac muscle

The smooth muscle

It is the muscle of the internal organs, e.g., the bladder, intestines. It has small spindle-shaped cells.

The individual cells are 2-5 µm in diameter and 40-200 µm in length. They do not have visible striations but they have myogenic activity.

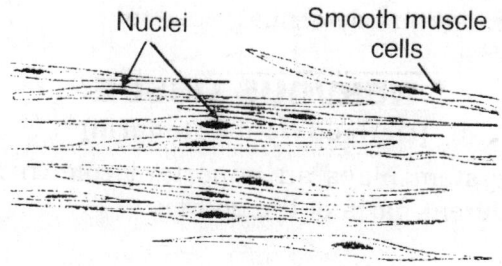

Fig. 2.6 Smooth muscle.

Each cell has a single nucleus. In addition, they contain cytoskeletal intermediate filaments which assist in the transmission of force generated during contraction to the neighboring smooth muscle cells and connective tissue. They also contain actin and myosin. They do not have any Z lines, but they have a functional counterpart that are distributed throughout the cytoplasm.

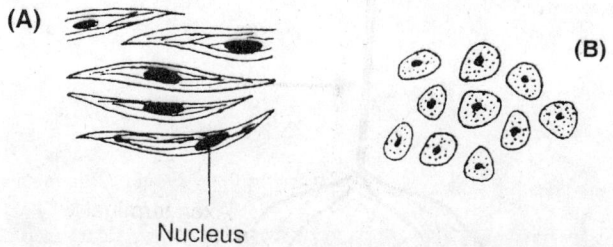

Fig. 2.7 A. Longitudiral section of smooth muscle. B. Horizontal section of smooth muscle.

The contractile protein filaments are attached to the *plasma membrane* at the junctional complex between the neighboring cells. Innervation to the smooth muscle is via autonomic nervous system.

Types

1. *Single unit* — Here the muscle fibers connect to one another by gap junctions and contract as a single unit; they are present in walls of hollow viscera, e.g., intestines, uninary bladder.
2. *Multi unit* — Multi unit smooth muscle fibers lack gap junctions and contract independently, e.g., blood vessels.

Both types of the smooth muscle are innervated by autonomic nervous system.

Tone is the steady level of tension maintained by a smooth muscle. The tone is under the control of following factors:

1. Circulating hormones
2. Local factors
3. Autonomic nervous system.

NERVOUS TISSUE
[Derived from Ectoderm]

The nervous system plays an important role in regulating the activities in different parts of the body.

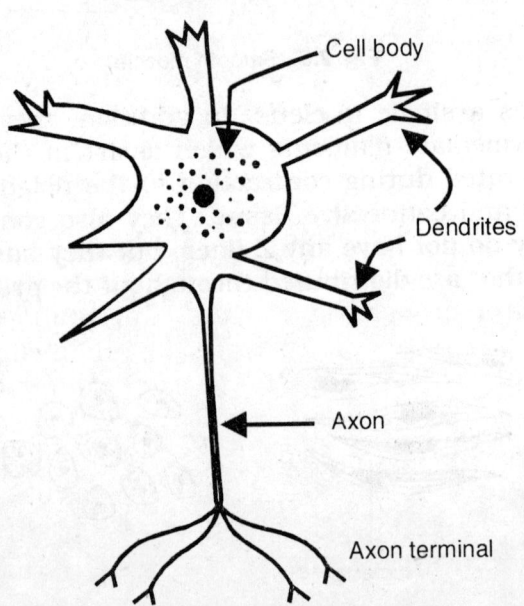

Fig. 2.8 A neuron can be unipular, bipolar or multipolar.

The organs of the nervous system are the brain, the spinal cord and the nerves.

Actual nervous tissue is ectodermal in origin. It has two types of cells :

1. *Nerve cells* — These are the conducting units of the system.
2. *Neuroglia* — These are connecting and supporting units.

Parts of neuron (Nerve cells) :

1. Soma — It is the cell body.
2. And two processes, one axon which transmit the nerve impulses away from the cell body and one or more dendrites which carry nerve signals towards the cell body.

Neuromuscular transmission

At the neuromuscular junction the nerve fibre branches at its end to form a complex of branching nerve terminals, which invaginate into the muscle fibre but lie outside the membrane. This entire structure is called *motor end plate*.

The invagination in the muscle membrane is known as *synaptic gutter*. The axon terminal contains many mitochondrias that supply ATP which is used for synthesis of acetylcholine, an excitatory transmitter.

On the inner surface of the neural membrane are linear dense bars; to each side of each dense bar are voltage gated Ca^{2+} channels. When an action potential spreads over the interior of the nerve terminal, the Ca^{2+} ions in turn exert an attractive influence on the acetylcholine vesicles, drawing them to the neural membrane adjacent to the dense bars. The vesicles then fuse with the neural membrane and empty their acetylcholine into the synaptic space by the process of exocytosis.

This acetylcholine gets bound to the acetylcholine receptors in the postsynaptic membrane leading to the opening of acetylcholine gated ion channels which allow the entry of Na^+, K^+ and Ca^{2+} to move easily through membrane. Thus large number of Na^+ ions move inside, creating a local positive potential change inside the muscle fibre membrane. This end plate potential initiates an action potential spreading along the muscle membrane and thus causes muscle contraction.

Polarisation in a nerve

Normally the nerve membrane is selectively permeable due to which Na^+ has the highest concentration in the ECF, while K^+ has about 30 fold more concentration within the cells. Due to this the inside is –ve as compared to outside and the potential difference is –70 mv.

When an impulse passes through an area of membrane then K^+ moves out and Na^+ moves in, thus reversing the polarity; this is known as depolarisation. Again the concentration is restored back to normal due to activity of Na^+–K^+ ATPase pump.

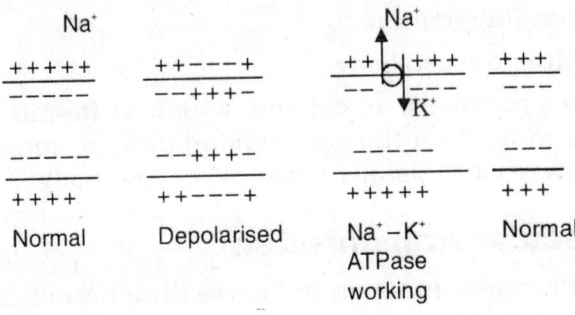

Fig. 2.9 Polarisation and depolarisation in a nerve.

Reaction of degeneration

Mature neurons are incapable of cell division. Therefore, damage to nervous tissue can be permanent. Nerves have a limited capacity to repair themselves. Stages of repair of an axon in a peripheral motor neuron are :

1. Following injury, distal portion of axon and myelin sheath degenerates.
2. Macrophages remove the debris.
3. Remaining neurilemma and endoneurium form a tunnel from the point of injury to the effector.
4. New Schwann cells grow in the tunnel to maintain a path for regrowth of the axon.
5. Cell body reorganizes its Nissl bodies to provide the needed proteins to extend the remaining healthy portion of the axon.
6. Axon sprouts appear.
7. When sprout reaches tunnel, its growth rate increases.
8. The skeletal muscle cell atrophies until the nervous connection is re-established.

3

BIO-CHEMICAL AND BIO-PHYSICAL PRINCIPLES

MATTER

Matter is anything which takes up space and posses mass. It has mass, weight and different states. Mass indicates the quantity of matter and is same everywhere, whereas weight indicates the force of attraction which the earth exerts on object. Matter exists in different states like solid, liquid and gaseous.

Construction of matter

Atoms — Atoms are the building block of matter. Structurally it is composed of neutron, proton and electron.

Neutrons — Neutrons are relatively heavy, electrically neutral and disintigrates into proton and an electron.

Protons — Protons are relatively heavy, carry a positive charge and its number, atomic number.

Electrons — Electrons are very light, carry a negative charge and move in shells around nucleus.

Mass number — Mass number is the number of neutrons and proton present in the nucleus.

Atomic mass — It is the combined mass of neutron and proton in the nucleus. Atomic mass is also calculated as relative atomic mass, using the relative mass of 12c as reference.

IONS

Ions are atoms which have lost or gained an electron. It is of two type — anion and cation. Anion are the atom which have gained an electron (–) where as cations are those atom which have lost an electron (+).

ISOTOPES

Isotopes are atom containing same number of proton, but differing in number of neutrons. It is of two types — stable and unstable. In stable isotopes very little decay occur whereas in unstable atoms decay via α particle emission, particle emission and ϒ radiation occurs.

Isotopes posses half life i.e. Ty^2 which is the time taken for half the atom present to decay.

Unstable isotopes are important diagnostically, therapeutically and pathogenically.

MOLECULES

These are the smallest amount of an element or compound which can exist alone and still exhibit the properties of the element or compound.

RADICLE

Group of atom which combine and behave like single ion.

COMPOUNDS

Compounds are those substances which are composed of two or more element and have combined chemically. These are of two types – *Inorganic* and *Organic*. Inorganic small molecules are good conductors of electricity while organic compounds are usually big molecules and poor conductors of electricity.

SALTS

These are the compounds composed of cation and anion. It is soluble in water and conduct electricity.

ELECTROLYTES

Electrolytes are those substance which dissociate into ion when dissolved in water and conduct electricity.

OSMOSIS

Osmosis can be defined as the net flow of solvent through a membrane which separtes the two solutions of different solute concentration.

It allows solvent molecules to pass through readily but prevents solute from passing through. Such a membrane is called selective permeable membrane.

Significance

Water constitutes about 60% of total body mass of an adult. Many solids are dissolved or colloidally dispersed in the body fluid. These substances are present in differing concentration. The water content of different compartments of the body tends to vary but it is stabilised by osmosis.

Purgatives, such as epsom salt (magnesium sulphate) act by increasing the flow of the water from the surrounding tissue spaces into the intestinal lumen. This results in increased fluidity of the intestinal contents hence facilitating bowel evacuation.

DIFFUSION

Diffusion is a process by which a gas or substance in solution moves or flows from region of higher concentration to region of lower concentration untill the concentration is uniform throughout both regions.

The extent of diffusion from one region to another is directly proportional to the difference in concentration in two regions and the cross-sectional areas across which diffusion is taking place and inversely proportional to the thickness of the boundary.

Features

1. Diffusion is a passive process — the particle supply the kinetic energy themselves.
2. Diffusion is affected by particle concentration, distance barrier and particle type.
3. In diffusion, it is the solute that moves.

Significance

Diffusion plays an important role in bodily functions. Nutrients are absorbed in the digestive tract by diffusion; oxygen and carbon dioxide are exchanged by diffusion.

Facilitated diffusion

Large molecules or molecules that are insoluble in cell membrane are transported across the membrane.

The molecules to be transported combine with special carrier molecules. This union creates a compound that is soluble in cell membrane and it can then diffuse through to the other side.

When this carrier-medicated transport takes place from an area of higher solute concentration to an area of lower concentration energy is not required and the process is called facilitated diffusion.

Examples :

1. Glucose transport by the glucose transporter across

intestinal epithelium.
2. The transport of glucose into RBC, muscle and adipose tissue in the presence of insulin.

FILTRATION

Filtration is the physical process by which water and solutes pass through a membrane when a hydrostatic pressure gradient exists across the membrane. Hydrostatic pressure is the force or weight of fluid pushing against the surface.

Filtration always takes place down a hydrostatic pressure gradient. This means that when two fluids have unequal hydrostatic pressures and are separated by a membrane, water and diffusible solute filter out of the solution that has the higher hydrostatic pressure.

Filtration differs from the Osmosis in that the water and solutes can filter or diffuse through a membrane where as by Osmosis only water can osmose through membrane.

Filtration is an important mechanism for moving substances through the walls of the blood capillaries.

CELLS

Cell is the fundamental unit of life. The three principle components of cells are :

1. Cell membrane.
2. Cytoplasm and it's organelles.
3. Nucleus and it's chromosomes.

Cell membrane

The cell membrane forms the outer boundary of the cell. It is more than a simple envelope for the cell. It is an actively functioning part of cell, an organelle in its own right.

Many chemical reactions take place within as well as on the surface of the membrane.

Functions of cell membrane :

1. It serves as a barrier between extracellular and intracellular compartments.
2. It is selectively permeable allowing only certain molecules through. The compositions at the extra and intracellular compartments therefore differ, e.g. the Na^+ and Ca^{2+} concentration are much higher extracellularly than intracellularly while the reverse is true for K^+ and mg^{2+}.

3. It is usually electrically charged or polarised.
4. It contains receptors, which bind hormones, neurotransmitters and drugs selectively.
5. It contain antigens, which activate the immune system —plays a major role in protection of the body and in disease process.

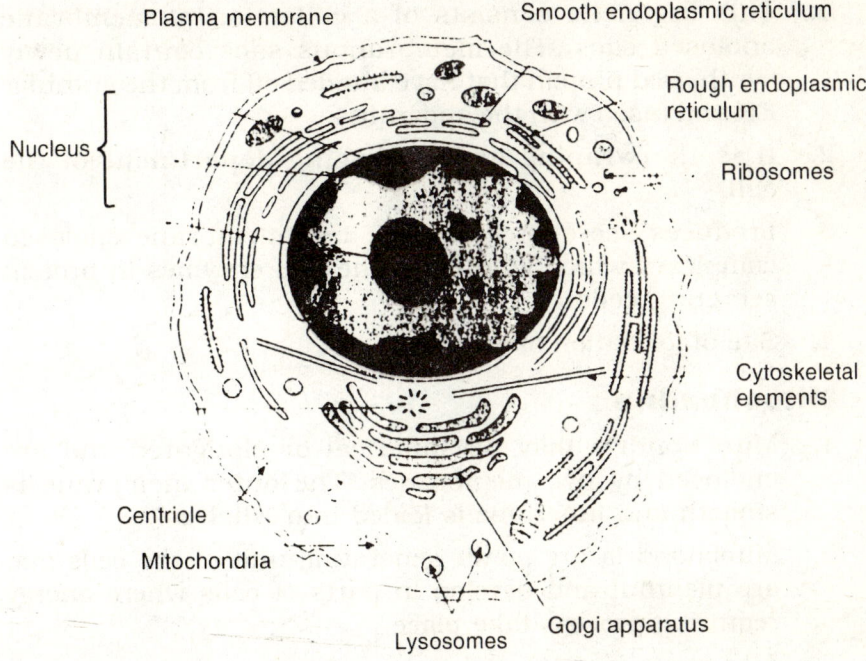

Fig. 3.1 Cell with its components.

Cytoplasm

The cytoplasm consists of semi fluid solution in which numerous subcellular permanent organelles are suspended.

The cytoplasm is the main area of the cell in which metabolic reactions take place. The organelles prevent these from interfering with one another as most reactions occur within the organelles.

Organelles

Endoplasmic reticulam : The E.R. consists of a network of fluid filled tubular canals distributed throughout the cytoplasm.

Types — Granular E.R. and Agranular E.R.

Granular ER — It is the site of protein synthesis.

It contain 65% RNA and 35% protein.

Ribosomes : Ribosomes are small bodies not surrounded by membrane and consisting of ribonucleo-protein. Free ribosomes tend to form chains called polyribosomes. The ribosomes attached to the ER synthesise proteins for cellular export.

Golgi apparatus :

1. This organelle consists of a collection of membrane enclosed sacs. The membranous sacs contain newly synthsised protein that have budded off from the granular ER and fused with the apparatus.
2. It is the wraping and packaging department of the cell.
3. Produces secretion granules, i.e., membrane enclosed complexes which store hormone and enzymes in protein secreting cells.
4. Site of formation of lysosomes.

Mitochondria :

1. Mitochondria may be spherical or elongated and are enclosed by two membranes. The outer membrane is smooth and inner one is folded into "shelves".
2. Mitochondria are power generating unit of the cells and are plentiful and develop in parts of cells where energy requiring process take place.
3. Also contains DNA and can synthesize protein.

Lysosomes : These are spherical or oval membrane-bounded bodies containing a variety of powerful enzymes. The lysosomes function as type of digestive system for the cell. Exogenous substances such as fragment of cells and bacteria that have been engulfed by particular cell, end up in membrane lined vacoule which fuse with lysosomes.

Enzymes bound in lysosomes include ribonuclease, deoxyribonuclease, phosphatase, collagenase and cathepsin.

Peroxisomes : These organelle are surrounded by a single membrane and are especially abundant in kidney and liver cells. They are involved in the production of hydrogen peroxide (H_2O_2) and one catalase that breaks H_2O_2 down to water. This is important as H_2O_2 is produced by many cells and is toxic.

Centrioles : In the cytoplasm of most cells are two cylindrical structures called centrioles. They are located near the nucleus and are arranged at right angles to each other.

The centrioles duplicate themselves at start of mitosis and are concerned with the movement of chromosomes during cell division.

Nucleus

Nucleus is found in most eukaryotic cells. The nucleus is the largest organelles and the cell usually contains only one nucleus with two membranes surrounding the nucleus.

The nucleus is mainly made up of chromosomes. Each chromosome is made up of a giant molecule of DNA almost completely covered by proteins of histone variety. The complex of DNA and protein is called chromatin.

The ultimate unit of heredity are the genes located on the chromosomes and each gene is a portion of the DNA molecules.

The nucleus directs cellular activity mainly by its production of several types of *nucleic acid*. These are in turn responsible for the synthesis of various protein enzymes that control cellular movements, growth and reproduction.

MITOSIS

Mitosis is the process of cell division where by a new cell is formed, containing hereditary information identical to that of the parent cell. This type of division occurs in all body cells apart from mature sex cells and is a most amazing phenomenon.

Five phases are distinguished in mitosis namely – interphase, prophase, metaphase, anaphase telophase.

Interphase

Chromosome not visible because they are unrolled in the form of long thin threads. The DNA replicates during this phase.

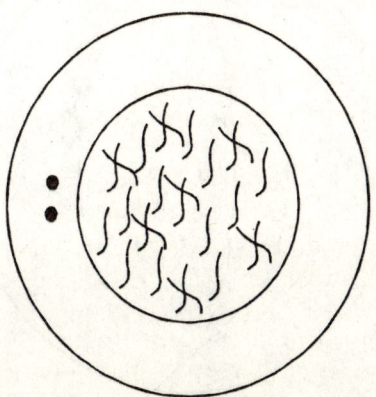

Fig. 3.2 Interphase.

Prophase

Centrioles move to opposite poles of cell forming the mitotic spindle between them. The nuclear membrane disintigrates. Chromatin becomes concentrated and visible as chromosomes. Each chromosome consists of two identical chromatids, held together at centromere. Microtubules appear.

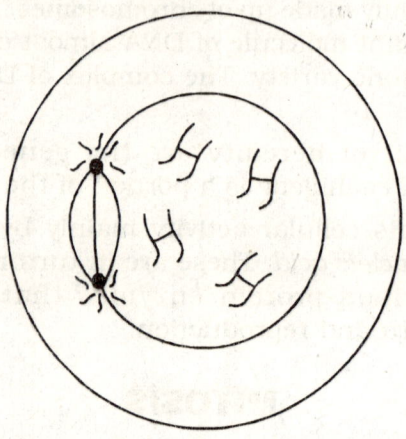

Fig. 3.3 Prophase.

Metaphase

Chromosomes line upon the equator of the spindle about midway between the centrioles and spindle fibres from both poles are attached to the centromere.

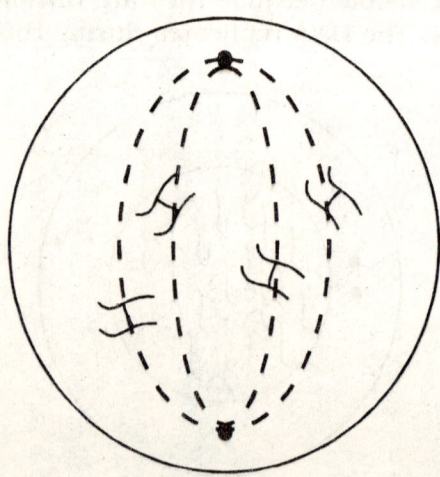

Fig. 3.4 Metaphase.

Anaphase

The chromosomes separate at the centromere and daughter chromosomes are pulled apart by the spindle fibres to opposite poles of the cell.

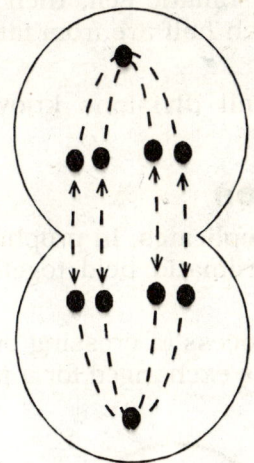

Fig. 3.5 Anaphase.

Telophase

The chromosomes reach the opposite poles; the spindle disappears. Nuclear membranes form around each group of chromosomes. A nucleolus appears in each newly formed nucleus, the cytoplasm is divided in the equitorial plane and two indentical daughter cells are formed. *Mitosis takes about two hour to be completed.*

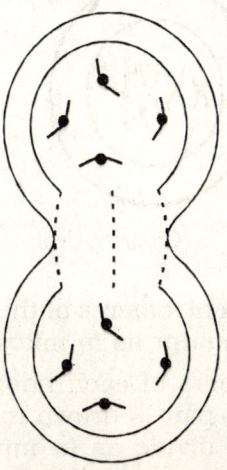

Fig. 3.6 Telophase.

MEIOSIS
[Division of sex cells]

Meiosis is a special kind of cell division which takes place during the formation of gametes in gonads. The aim of meiosis is to reduce the number of chromosomes in a cell by half.

The fertilised ovum like somatic cell, then contains 46 chromosomes or 23 pairs of which half are from father and half from the mother.

Meiosis includes two cell divisions known as *meiosis I* and *meiosis II*.

First meiotic division

During interphase DNA replicates. In prophase the chromosomes, each consting of two chromatid held together by a centromere, become visible.

During this phase the process of crossing over occurs, whereby a part of one chromosome is exchanged for a part of another.

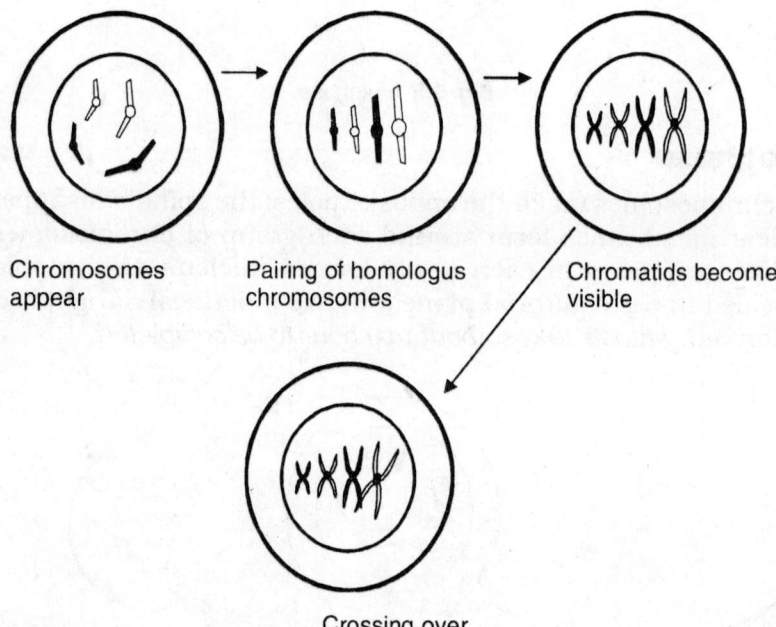

Chromosomes appear   Pairing of homologus chromosomes   Chromatids become visible

Crossing over

During metaphase the centromeres of the chromosomal pairs align themselves along the equator as in mitosis.

In anaphase, the members of each homologus chromosome pair split and one from each pair is drawn to opposite pole of the cell. The centromere do not divide as in mitosis and the number of chromosomes that move to opposite pole of the cell is therefore the half the normal number.

In telophase, cleavage of the cytoplasm occurs and formation of two daughter cells, each containing a haploid number of chromosomes, is completed.

Second meiotic division

This follows almost immediately after the 1st division. The centromeres divide and duplicate chromosomes separate. Thus two daughter cells each with a haploid number of chromosomes and each containing one chromatid are formed from each of the previous two daughter cells. Altogether four haploid cells are thus formed during meiosis.

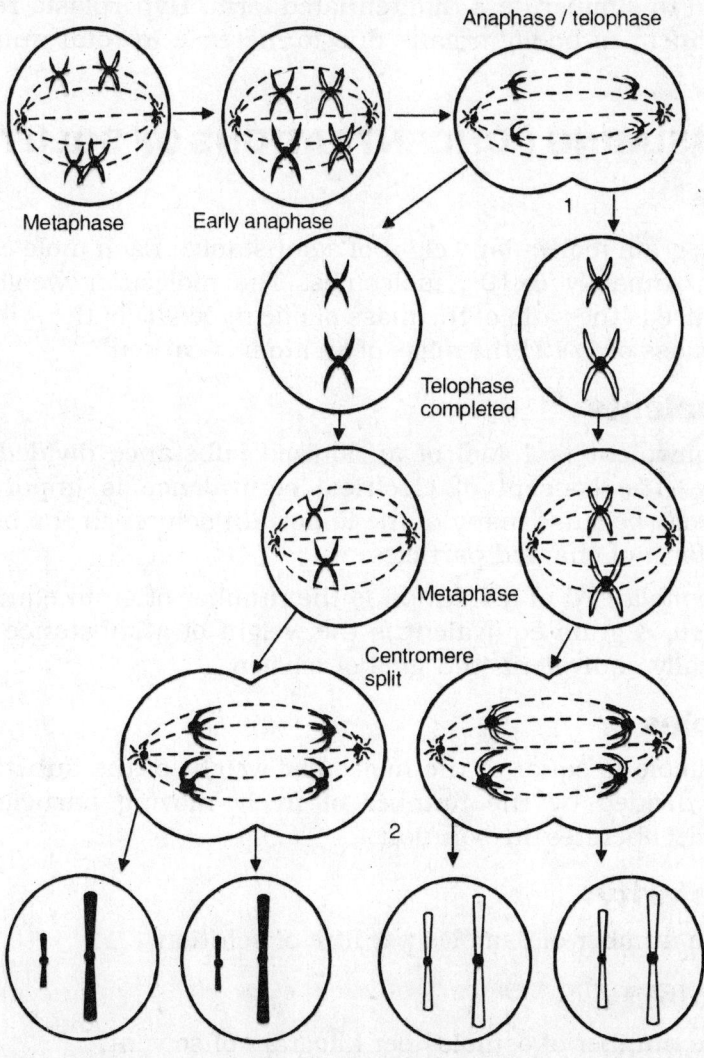

Fig. 3.7 Meiosis

CANCER

Cancer may be defined as condition of uncontrolled reproduction of cells. Cells do not respond to or obey the normal mitotic control mechanism. As a result, cancer cells eventually give rise to a large cell population.

Cancer cells often get detached from the cellular mass and may be carried away from the site of origin to establish new cancerous growth elsewhere in the body which is known as metastasis. Metastasis is characteristic of cancer.

The terms anaplasia and hyperplasia are associated with cancer. Anaplasia refers to condition where particular animal cells have reverted to simpler, less differentiated form. Hyperplasia refers to enlargement of bodily organs due to increase in total number of cells.

MEASURING CONCENTRATIONS OF SOLUTION

Moles

It is the gram molecular weight of a substance. Each mole consists of approximately 6×10^{23} molecules. The molecular weight of a substance is the ratio of the mass of one molecule of the substance to the mass of $1/12^{th}$ the mass of an atom of carbon^{12}.

Equivalents

One equivalent is 1 Mol of an ionized substance divided by its valency. The concept of electrical equivalence is important in physiology because many of the important solutes in the body are in the form of charged particles.

The *Normality* (N) of a solution is the number of gram equivalents in 1 litre. A gram equivalent is the weight of a substance that is chemically equivalent to 8 gms of oxygen.

Osmoles

One osmole is equal to the molecular weight of the substance in grams divided by the number of freely moving particles each molecule liberates in solution.

Osmolarity

It is the number of osmoles per litre of solution.

Osmolality

It is the number of osmoles per kilogram of solvent.

Osmolarity is affected by the volume of the various solutes in the solution and the temperature, while osmolality is not.

Osmolal concentration of a substance in a fluid is measured by the degree to which it depresses the freezing point. It is expressed as osmoles per liter of water.

IONS

Ions are the substances which are present in the charged state in the body.

The main ions in the body include Na^+, K^+, Cl^-, Ca^{2+}, proteins etc. The concentration of Na^+ is approximately 10 times outside the cell as compared to inside. While that of K^+ is about greater than 20 times more inside as compared to outside. Cl^- is also more outside the cell as compared to inside of the cell.

These ions perform various functions like:
1. Maintaining the membrane potentials.
2. Intercellular communication.
3. Excitation of nerves and conduction of impulses.
3. Contraction of the muscles.
4. Maintaining various reflexes in the body like tendon, etc.
5. Balancing energy production, metabolism and other functions.

ELECTROLYTES

These are the substances which get dissociated into their ions in the aqueous state, e.g. Na^+, K^+, Cl^-, HCo_3^- etc.

The main electrolytes of human body are NaCl and proteins which get converted into Na^+, Cl^- and Pro^-. Other examples are KCl, $NaHCo_3$, etc.

These help in various functions in body (as noted above in ions). But they are very useful for diagnosing a disease condition since they get altered from the normal values.

For example, in patients with adrenocortical diseases the concentration of Na^+ and Cl^- in plasma gets lowered while that of k^+ gets increased.

NON-ELECTROLYTES

These are the substances which do not dissociate into their ions when dissolved in the aqueous solutions.

For example, Glucose, Urea.

These are mainly the substances which take part in various metabolic reactions or which are waste products. The assessment of the concentration of these substances also provide various information about the disease.

For e.g. increase in the concentration of uric acid in plasma above 7 mg% is a condition known as hyperuricemia, which leads to the formation of gout sometimes.

FILTERATION

It is the process by which fluid is forced through a membrane or other barrier because of a difference in pressure on the two sides.

The amount of fluid filtered in a given interval is proportionate to the difference in pressure, the surface area of the membrane and the permeability of the membrane. It is an important phenomenon in the body functioning; *for example*, in kidney the function is to filter out waste products from the blood.

ABSORPTION

It is defined as the taking up of a substance. Like the filteration, absorption is also an important function of the body. The substances which are broken down into simpler particles are taken up and used in the body by the help of absorption.

The substances like vitamins, minerals and water cross the mucosa and enter the lymph or the blood.

Active absorption

This type of absorption requires energy.

E.g. the absorption of Glucose, when the last traces are not absorbed passively. Cl^- is also an example.

Passive absorption

In this type of absorption no energy is required.

E.g. absorption of Na^+, K^+, H_2O.

DONAN EQUILIBRIUM

According to this concentration of +vely charged ions is slightly greater in the plasma than in the interstitial fluid.

This effect is due to plasma proteins which have a net negative charge and therefore tend to bind cations like Na^+ and K^+. Thus, holding extra amounts of these in the plasma with the plasma proteins.

ACIDS

These are substances that are capable of donating protons. E.g. HCL, H_2CO_3. Strong acids dissociate completely while weak acids ionize incompletely.

COLLOIDS

There are the substances which have a high molecular weight but are present in large amounts.

E.g. Plasma proteins.

These are unable to cross the apertures in the wall of capillaries. Thus they exert a pressure from inside of capillaries on the fluid present outside, thus pulling it inside.

The colloid osmotic pressure due to the plasma colloids is called the oncotic pressure.

SURFACE TENSION

It is the property due to which the surface tries to acquire minimum surface area. This is an important factor in the lungs since it affects the respiration. Because when greater is the surface tension lesser will be the air inspired due to increased friction.

In order to decrease this the surfactant plays a major role. It has dipalmitoyl phosphatidyl choline which reduces the surface tension.

BASES

These are substances which are capable of accepting a proton.

The normal pH of the plasma is 7.4. If pH is below 7.35, it is called acidosis which is also defined as accumulation of acid while accumulation of base is known as alkalosis.

Normal pH of blood : Arterial → 7.35 – 7.45

Venous → 7.31 – 7.41

ENZYMES

They are biologic polymers that catalyze multiple dynamic processes, which make life as we know, possible. As the determinants of rates at which physiologic events take place, enzymes play central role in health and disease. Enzymes are classified by reaction type and mechanism. IUB system of classification of enzyme is :

1. Reactions and the enzymes that catalyze them form six classes.
2. The enzyme name has two parts. The first names the substrate or substrates. The second ending in – ase indicates the type of reaction catalyzed. Additional information, if needed to clarify the reaction, may follow in parenthesis, for e.g. the enzyme catalysing L-melate +NAD^+ $\rightleftharpoons$ pyruvate +CO_2 +NADH +H^+ is designated 1.1.1. 37L – malate: NAD^+ oxidoreductase.

3. Each enzyme has a code no. (EC) that characterizes the reaction type as to class (first digit), subclass (second digit), subsubclass (third digit). The fourth digit is for specific enzyme. Many enzymes require a coenzyme. Coenzymes that are tightly associated with an enzyme through either covalant bonding or non-covalant bonding form the prosthetic groups.

Properties of enzymes

1. Like other proteins, enzymes get denatured at high temperature, so they are thermolabile.
2. Enzyme molecules can exist as simple proteins or can combine with metal ions to form metalloproteins or form conjugate proteins.
3. Most of the enzymes require co-enzymes or co-factors for activity.
4. They combine with substrate to from enzyme substrate complex, which can lower the energy of activation.

$$E + S \longleftrightarrow ES \longleftrightarrow E + P$$

5. They posses active sites at which the substrate binds to form enzyme substrate complex.
6. They do not alter the reaction equilibrium.
7. They are specific for substrates.

Almost all enzymes are proteins and act as biocatalysts. Exception is ribozyme, a ribonucleotide which catalyses cleavage and joining of RNA molecule.

4

PROTEINS, CARBOHYDRATES AND LIPIDS

PROTEINS

Proteins are the most abundant and essential organic molecules. These are polymers of *Amino Acids.*

Amino acids

Essential	Non-Essential
Lysine	Alanine
Isoleucine	Asparagine
Leucine	Aspartate
Methionine	Cysteine
Threonine	Glutamate
Valine	Glutamine
Phenylalanine	Glycine
Tryptophan	Hyoroxyproline
	Proline
	Serine
	Tyrosine

Structural classification :
1. With Aliphatic side chains
    - (a) Glycine
    - (b) Alanine
    - (c) Valine
    - (d) Leucine
    - (e) Isoleucine

2. With Hydroxyl group
   (a) Serine
   (b) Threonine
   (c) Tyrosine
3. With Sulphur
   (a) Cysteine
   (b) Methionine
4. Acidic AA
   (a) Aspartic acid
   (b) Asparagine
   (c) Glutamic acid
   (d) Glutamine
5. Basic AA
   (a) Argenine
   (b) Lysine
   (c) Histidine
6. Aromatic AA
   (a) Histidine
   (b) Phenylalanine
   (c) Tyrosine
   (d) Tryptophan
7. Imino acids
   (a) Proline

CARBOHYDRATES

Carbohydrates may be defined as polyhydroxyaldehydes or ketones or compounds which produce them on hydrolysis.

They are primarily composed *of carbon, hydrogen and oxygen.*

Carbohydrates are classified into four groups :

Monosaccharides

1. These are simplest form of carbohydrates.
2. General formula : $C_n(H_2O)_n$.
3. They cannot be further hydrolysed.

Proteins, carbohydrate and lipids

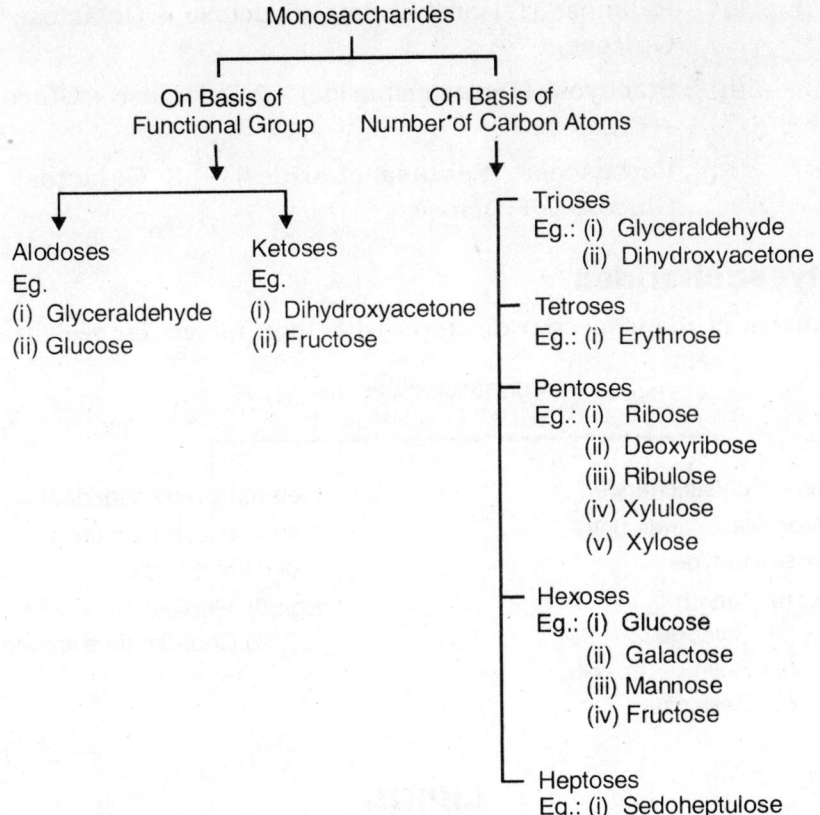

Disaccharides

1. General Formula : $C_n(H_2O)_{n-1}$
2. On hydrolysis, these produce two molecules of same or different monosaccharides.

   Eg.: (i) Maltose (Glucose + Glucose)

   (ii) Sucrose (Glucose + Fructose)

   (iii) Lactose (Glucose + Galactose)

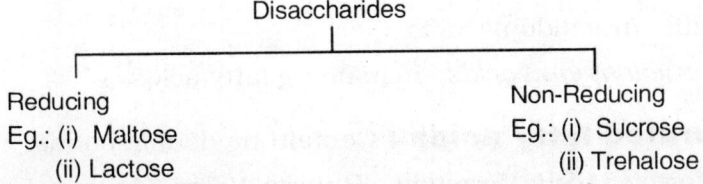

Oligosaccharides

1. These contain more than two monosaccharide molecules.
2. General formula : $C_n(H_2O)_{n-1}$

Eg.: (i) Raffinose (Trisaccharide) – Fructose + Galactose + Glucose.

(ii) Stachyose (Tetrasaccharide) – 2 Galactose + Glucose + Fructose

(iii) Verbascose (Pentasaccharides) – 3 Galactose + Glucose + Fructose

Polysaccharides

Polymers of monosaccharide units with high molecular weight.

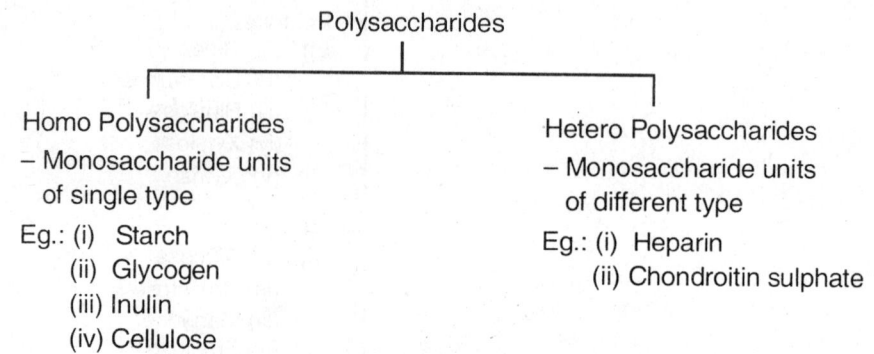

Polysaccharides

Homo Polysaccharides
– Monosaccharide units of single type
Eg.: (i) Starch
(ii) Glycogen
(iii) Inulin
(iv) Cellulose

Hetero Polysaccharides
– Monosaccharide units of different type
Eg.: (i) Heparin
(ii) Chondroitin sulphate

LIPIDS

Lipids may be regarded as organic substances relatively insoluble in water but soluble in organic solvents.

Simple lipids

Fats : Esters of fatty acids with Glycerol.

Essential fatty acids : Mainly pufa (Poly-unsaturated-fatty-acids)

Eg.: (i) Linoleic acid
(ii) Linolenic acid
(iii) Arachidonic acid

Non-essential fatty acids : Remaining fatty acids.

Saturated fatty acids : Contain no double bonds.

Eg.: Formic, Acetic, Propionic, Butyric, Valric, (Aproic), Lauric, Palmtic, Stearic, Arachidic.

Unsaturated Fatty Acids : Contain one or more double bonds.

(i) Monounsaturated

   Eg.:- Monoethenoid and Monoenoic

(ii) Polyunsaturated

   Eg.:- Polyethnoid, Polyenoic

(iii) Eicosanoids

   Eg.:- Prostanoids, Leukotrienes, Lipoxins.

Waxes : Esters of fatty acids with higher molecular weight; monohydric alcohols.

Complex lipids

Esters of fatty acids with alcohol, containing additional groups.

Phospholipids : Contain additional phosphoric acid residue.

Eg.: (i) Glycero Phospholipids

(ii) Phosphatidic acid

(iii) Lecithin

(iv) Cephalins

(v) Phosphatidylinositol

(vi) Cardiolipin

Glycolipids Contain additional phosphonic acid residue. Cerebrocides are simplest form of glycolipids.

Other complex lipids :

Eg.: (i) Sulfolipids

(ii) Aminolipids

Derived lipids

Eg.: (i) Fatty acids

(ii) Glycerol

(iii) Steroids

(iv) Alcohols

(v) Fatty aldehydes

(vi) Ketone bodies

vii) Hormones

Neutral lipids

They are uncharged.

Eg.: (i) Acylglycerols
 (ii) Cholesterol
 (iii) Cholesteryl esters

5

NUTRITION AND HEALTH

INTRODUCTION

Nutrition may be defined as the science of food and its relation to health.

CLASSIFICATION OF FOOD

1. **Classification by origin**
   - (a) Foods of animal origin
   - (b) Foods of plant origin

2. **Classification by chemical composition**
   - (a) Proteins
   - (b) Fats
   - (c) Carbohydrates
   - (d) Vitamins
   - (e) Minerals

3. **Classification by predominant function**
   - (a) Body building foods
   - (b) Energy giving foods
   - (c) Protective foods

4. **Classification by nutritive value**
   - (a) Cereals and millets
   - (b) Pulses
   - (c) Vegetables
   - (d) Nuts and oilseeds
   - (e) Fruits
   - (f) Animal food

(g) Fat and oils
(h) Sugar and jaggery
(i) Condiments and spices
(j) Miscellaneous food

NUTRIENTS

These are organic and inorganic complexes contained in food, each having some specific function.

These are of 2 types :

1. Macro nutrients – Form main bulk of food (include Proteins, Fats and Carbohydrates).
2. Micro nutrients – Minerals and vitamins.

PROTEINS

Proteins are polymers of amino acids and contain C, H, O, N and S (Required 1 gm/kg of body wt. daily).

Functions

1. Body building.
2. Repair and maintenance of body tissues.
3. Osmotic pressure.
4. Synthesis of different compounds.
5. Supply energy.

Sources

1. Animal sources – Milk, meat, egg, cheese, fish.
2. Vegetable sources – Pulses, cereals, beans, nuts.

Metabolism

1. They are not stored and have to be replaced.
2. They are constantly under turnover i.e. being broken down and reused.
3. Both amount and pattern of specific protein are maintained in body.

Assessment of protein nutrition status

Following tests are done :

1. Arm muscle circumference.
2. The creatinine-height index.

3. Serum albumin and transferrin.
4. Total body nitrogen.

FATS

Fats are solid at 20 °C; if liquid they are called oils.

Classification
1. Simple lipids – Triglycerides.
2. Compound lipids – Phospholipids.
3. Derived lipids – Cholesterol.

Fatty Acids are product of fat hydrolysis and are of 2 types:
1. Saturated
2. Unsaturated

Sources
1. Animal fats – Ghee, butter, milk, cheese, meat.
2. Vegetable fats – Groundnut, mustard, coconut.
3. Other – Cereals, pulses, nuts.

Functions
1. Provide energy and are storehouse of energy.
2. Vehicle for fat soluble vitamins.
3. Provide support to viscera.
4. Beneath skin it provide insulation.
5. For body growth.

Diseases
1. Obesity
2. Phrenoderma
3. Coronary heart diseases
4. Cancer
5. Others like kwashiorkor

Requirement
30-40% of total energy intake.

CARBOHYDRATE

Main source of energy (4 Kcal/gm) and essential for oxidation of fats.

Present as starch, sugar and cellulose.

VITAMINS

Vitamins may be classified as :
1. Fat soluble vitamins (Vit. A, D, E, K).
2. Water soluble vitamins (Vit. B complex, C)

Vitamin A (Retinol)

Retinol, Pro-vitamin and B-Carotene.

Functions :
1. For normal vision
2. For normal functioning of glandular and epithelial tissue
3. Anti-infective

Sources :
1. Animal – Liver, egg, butter, cheese, milk, fish and meat.
2. Plant – Green leafy vegetables.

Deficiency causes :
1. Xerophthalmia (Dry eye)
2. Keratomalacia
3. Night blindness
4. Bitot's spots
5. Corneal xerosis
6. Conjunctival xerosis

Toxicity by excessive intake.

Vitamin D (Colecalciferol Vit. D_5) (Califerol – Vit. D_2) (Kidney Hormone)

Stored in fat depots.

Functions :
1. Absorption of Calcium and Phosphorus.
2. Stimulates normal mineralisation of bones.
3. Permits normal growth.

Sources :
1. Sunlight – by UV rays.
2. Foods – Liver, egg, butter.

Deficiency causes :
1. Rickets – in children.
2. Osteomalacia – in adults.

Vitamin E (Tocopherol)
1. α –Tocopherol is biologically most potent.
2. Sources – Vegetable oils, cotton seed, sunflower seed.

Vitamin K (Major forms – Vit. K_1 & K_2)
1. Sources – Green vegetables, cow's milk and human milk.
2. It is stored in liver.
3. In deficiency blood clotting time is increased.
4. Requirement is met by dietary intake and microbial synthesis in gut.

Thiamine (Vit. B_1) (Water Soluble)
1. Sources – All natural foods.
2. Thiamine is lost on processing of rice and wheat.

Deficiency :
1. Peripheral neuritis
2. Cardiac beri-beri
3. Infantile beri-beri
4. Wernicke's encephalopathy in Alcoholics

Riboflavin (Vit. B_2) (Role in cellular oxidation)
Sources : Milk, egg, liver, kidney and green leafy vegetables.

Deficiency causes :
1. Ariboflavinosis
2. Angular stomatitis, cheilosis and glossitis.

Niacin (Nicotinic acid)
1. Essential for metabolism of carbohydrates, fats and proteins.
2. Sources – Liver, kidney, meat, poultry, fish, ground-nut.

Deficiency causes : Pellagra — diarrhoea, dermatitis and dementia.

Vitamin-B_6 (Pyridoxine)
1. Three forms: Pyridoxine, pyridoxal and pyridoxamine.
2. Important role in amino acid, fat and carbohydrate metab.

Sources : Milk, liver, meat, egg, fish, cereals.

Deficiency is associated with peripheral neuritis.

Pantothenic acid

1. Role in corticosteroid synthesis.
2. Present in cells as COA.

Folate (Folacin)

Occurs as free or bound folates.

Sources : Liver, meat, egg, milk.

Deficiency : Megaloblastic anaemia, glossitis, cheilosis.

Vitamin-B_{12}

Absorption requires intrinsic factor.

Deficiency :
1. Megaloblastic anemia (Pernicious).
2. Neurological lesions.

Vitamin C (Ascorbic acid)

Functions :
1. In tissue oxidation.
2. Needed for formation of collagen.

Sources : Citrus fruits.

Deficiency : Scurvy.

Calcium (Serum Ca^{++} level : 9-11 mg%)

Functions :
1. Formation of bones and teeth.
2. Coagulation of blood.
3. Contraction of muscles.
4. Relay of electric messages.

Sources : Milk and milk products.

Deficiency : No clear cut disease.

Phosphorus

1. Essential for formation of bones and teeth.
2. Deficiency is rare.
3. Widely distributed in food.

Sodium
1. Found in all body fluids.
2. Loss thorugh urine can be regulated by kidney but not sweat.

Potassium
Occurs widely in food and deficiency is rare.

Magnesium
1. Constituent of bones and present in all cells.
2. Essential for normal metabolism.

Iron

Functions :
1. In Hb (Haemoglobin).
2. Brain development and function.
3. Regulation of body temperature, muscle activity.
4. T cell production.

Sources :
1. Liver, meat, poultry and fish, cereals, green leafy vegetables.
2. Iron is absorbed in ferrous state in duodenum and upper small intestine and uptake is affected by presence of inhibitors and promoters.

Iron Losses : Haemorrage, basal losses.

Deficiency causes :
1. Anaemia (Microcytic).
2. Impaired immunity.

Evaluation of iron status :
1. Hb concentration.
2. Serum iron concentration.
3. Serum ferritin.
4. Serum transferrin.
5. Bone marrow iron.

Iodine
In thyroid hormones T_3 and T_4.

Sources : Sea food, Iodised salt.

Deficiency : Iodine deficiency disorders
1. Goitre.
2. Hypothyroidism.
3. Retarded physical and mental growth.
4. Cretinism.

Fluorine
Found in bones and teeth.

Sources : Drinking H_2O and foods

Two edged sword :
1. Deficiency – Dental caries.
2. Excess – fluorosis.

Zinc
1. Component of many enzymes.
2. Present in all tissues.
3. Widely distributed in food stuff.

Copper
1. Widely distributed.
2. Deficiency rare.
3. Wilson's disease.

Cobalt
1. Part of Vit. B12.
2. Deficiency may cause goitre.

Chromium
There are unusual glucose tolerance curve in response to chromium which suggests its role in carbohydrate metabolism.

Molybdenum
Excess : Bony deformities.

Deficiency : Mouth and oesophageal cancer.

Selenium
1. Selenium deficiency occurs in protein energy malnutrition.
2. Selenium + Vit. E deficiency reduces antibody production.

6

THE BLOOD

INTRODUCTION

The blood consist of cells and plasma.

COMPOSITION

1. Cells (46%)
   (a) R.B.C. (Red blood cells)
   (b) W.B.C. (White blood cells)
   (c) Platelets
2. Plasma (54%)
   (a) 9% solids

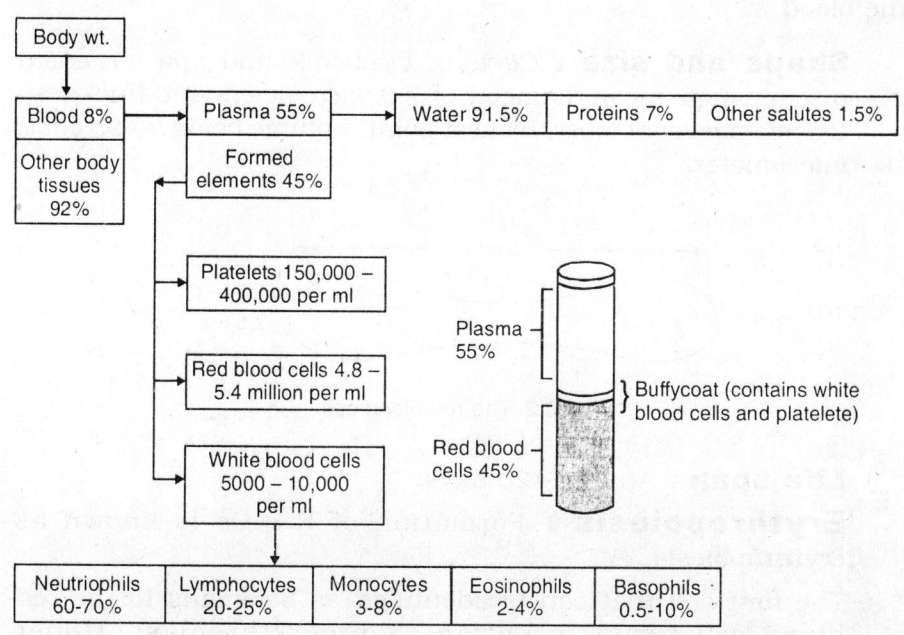

Fig. 6.1 Composition of blood.

(i) *Organic*
- Proteins
- Other substances

(ii) *Inorganic*
- Na^+, K^+, HCO_3^-, Cl^-
- Ca^{2+}, Fe^{2+}, Fe^{3+}

(b) 91% water

If blood clots then the retracted clot gives out serum.

Therefore, Serum = Plasma – (Fibrinogen and clotting factor)

Specific gravity of blood : 1050-1060

Volume of blood = 5-6 liters

BLOOD CELLS

R.B.C. (Erythrocytes)

R.B.C. contains haemoglobin, which in turn carries oxygen from the lungs to the tissues. They also contain large quantity of carbonic anhydrase, which catalyses the reversible reaction between carbon dioxide and water, increases the rate of this reaction to several thousand times. The haemoglobin in the cells is an excellent buffer making the red cells to act as the best acid-base buffering power of the blood.

Shape and size : *Circular, biconcave* and *non nucleated disc* having a mean diameter of *7.8 micrometers* and thickness *2.5 micrometer* at most thickest point. Volume being *90-95 cubic micrometers*.

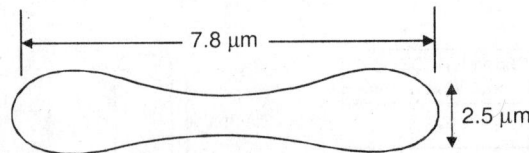

Fig. 6.2 The red blood cell.

Life span : Around 120 days.

Erythropoiesis : Formation of R.B.Cs is known as erythropoiesis.

The first cell that can be identified as belonging to the red blood cell series is knwon as proerythroblast. Under appropriate stimulation, this is then converted to basophil erythroblast and then as shown in the following figure to polychromatophil erythroblast, orthochromatic erythroblast, reticulocyte, and erythrocyte subsequently.

Proerythroblast
↓
Basophil erythroblast
↓
Polychromatophil erythroblast
↓
Orthochromatic erythroblast
↓
Reticulocytes
↓
Erythrocytes

Composition of R.B.C. :

1. 62% water.
2. 35% haemoglobin.
3. 3% other.

Production of blood cells : Development of blood cells is known as hemopoiesis. For R.B.Cs erythropoisis is the term used.

The pleuripotent haemopoitic stem cells are present in bone marrow. Production of blood cells in bone marrow continues throughout life. Some of the lymphocytic precursor stem cells migrate to thymus and produce T-lymphocytes wheares the others remaining in the bone marrow and produce B-Lymphocytes. Multipotent stem cells present in marrow give rise to committed stem cells responsible for production of different blood cells lines.

Erythropoiesis regulation : Hypoxia causes the kidney and the liver to secrete erythropoietin which in turn stimulates proerythroblast and leads to erythropoiesis.

Note : Intrinsic factor (IF) + extrinsic factor together forms Haematinic principle.

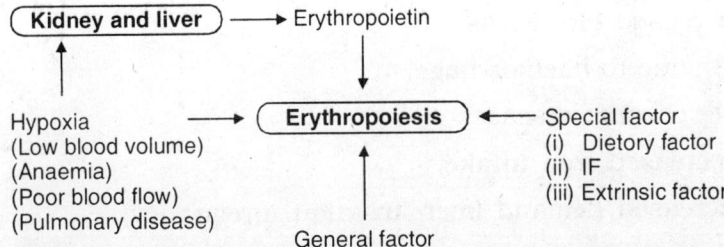

ANAEMIAS

Anaemia is reduction in haemoglobin content to less than 12 gm% or the number of R.B.Cs to less than 4 million/mm³ of blood. Anaemia can be blood loss anaemia, aplastic anaemia, megaloblastic anaemia or haemolytic anaemia.

Wintrobe's classification of Anaemia

	Normochromic	Hypochromic
Normocytic	Normocytic Normochromic	Hypochromic Normocytic
Macrocytic	Normochromic Macrocytic	Hypochromic Macrocytic
Microcytic	Normochromic Microcytic	Hypochromic Microcytic

Normocytic	—	Normal size
Macrocytic	—	Large size
Microcytic	—	Small size
Normochromic	—	Normal haemoglobin contents
Hypochromic	—	Less haemoglobin contents

Addison's anaemia

Due to lack of intrinsic factor with subsequent failure in absorption of Vit. B_{12}.

Folic acid deficiency anaemia

Folic acid deficiency produces anaemia.

Iron deficiency anaemia

It is the commonest anaemia in India. It's causes are :

1. Increased blood loss
   (a) due to haemorrhage
   (b) chronic diseases
2. Decreased iron intake.
3. Increased demand (menstruation, pregnancy).
4. Disturbance in iron utilization properly.

WHITE BLOOD CELLS OR W.B.C. OR LEUCOCYTES

W.B.C. are the mobile units of the body protective system. Formation of W.B.Cs take place in bone marrow and lymphoid tissue.

W.B.C. are *20,000/mm³* at birth and decrease to *4000-11000/mm³* in adults. The W.B.C. consist of following types of cells :

1. Polymorphonuclear neutrophil   62%
2. Polymorphonuclear eosinophil   2.3%
3. Polymorphonuclear basophil   0.4%
4. Monocytes   5.3%
5. Lymphocytes   30%

Polymorphonuclear neutrophils – (62%)

Phagocytosis. They have defence properties. Neutrophils act as first line of defence against bacterial infection. Neutrophils move by diapedesis through the capillary pores and by chemotaxis towards an area damaged by the invasive organism.

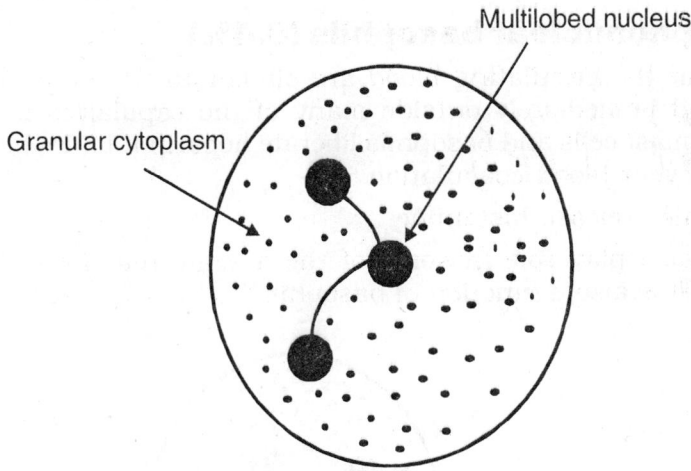

Besides being the first line defence the polymorphonuclear neutrophils also contain fever producing substances.

Applied Physiology : Neutropenia means decrease in neutrophils (infancy or viral infection).

Neutrophilia means increase in neutrophils (exercise, injury or pyogenic infection).

Polymorphonuclear eosinophils (2-3%)

They also act in *phagocytosis.*

- *Allergic reaction* – Eosinophils collect at the site of allergic reaction and limit their intensity.
- *Hypersensitivity* – They also participate in hypersensitivity reactions.

Applied : Eosinophilia – Increase in eosinophils.

Eosinopenia – Decrease in eosinophils.

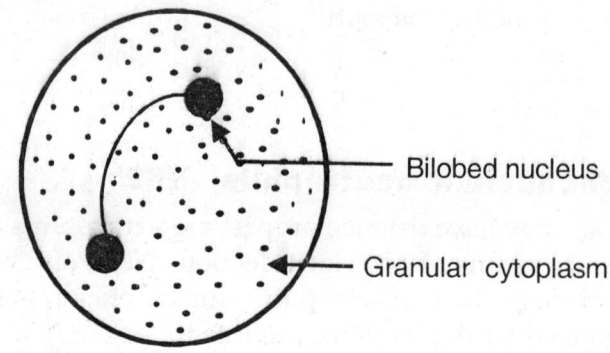

Polymorphonuclear basophils (0.4%)

Basophils in the circulating blood are similar to the large mast cells located immediately outside many of the capillaries in the body. Both mast cells and basophils liberate heparin into the blood. Heparin prevent blood coagulation.

Basophils also release histamine.

Basophils also play role in some of the allergic reactions. Mild phagocytosis is also a function of basophils.

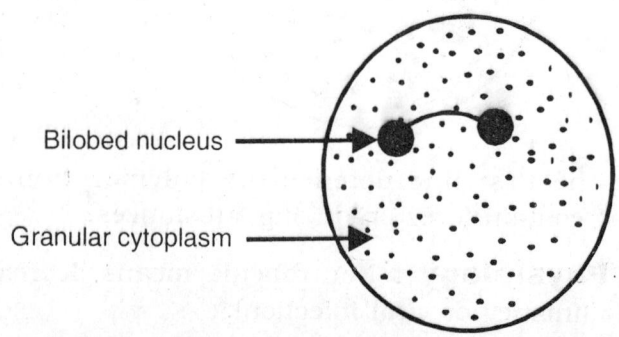

Applied physiology :

Basophilia – Increase in basophils as seen in T.B., chikenpox.

Basopenia – Decrease in basophils.

Monocytes (5.3%)

Monocytes come next to neutrophils in *phagocytosis*.

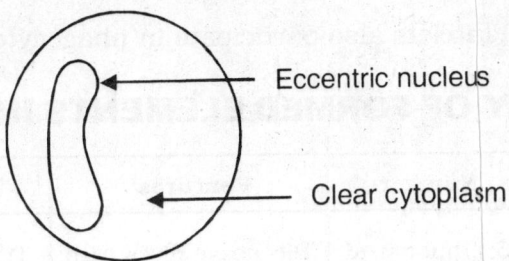

Monocytes *kill tumour cells* after sensitization by lymphocyte.

Applied physiology :

Monocytosis – Increase in monocytes as seen in T.B., syphilis.

Monocytopenia – Decrease in monocytes as seen in hypoplastic bone marrow.

Lymphocytes

1. Antibodies production.
2. Lymphocytes are of two types — small and large.

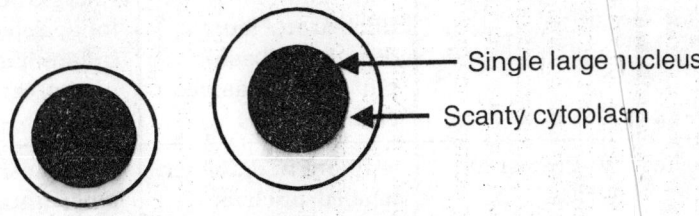

Small lymphocyte   Large lymphocyte

Applied physiology :

Lymphocytosis – Increase in lymphocytes as seen in chronic infective condition.

Lymphopenia – Decrease in lymphocytes as seen in AIDS.

PLATELETS

Platelets are the smallest blood cells. They are 2-4 lacs/mm^3 in count.

Development

Development of platelets is known as *thrombopoiesis*.

Functions

Haemostasis – Bleeding arrest. Platelets play a major role in blood haemostasis.

Phagocytosis – Platelets also participate in phagocytosis.

SUMMARY OF FORMED ELEMENTS IN BLOOD

Cell type	Number	Features	Functions
Red blood cells	~ 5.4 million/µl in males and ~ 4.8 million/µl in females.	Biconcave discs with diameter of 7-8 µm. Lifespan – 120 days.	Transport of oxygen and carbon dioxide in blood.
Neutrophils	60-70% of all WBCs.	2-5 lobed nucleus; 10-12 µm in diameter – fine cytoplasmic granules.	Phogocytosis; kills bacteria.
Eosinophils	2-4% of all WBCs.	Size – 10-12 µm diameter; bilobed nuclus; large eosinophilic granules.	Allergic reactions; action against parasitic worms.
Basophils	0.5-1% of all WBCs.	8-10 µm in diameter. Bilobed nucleus; deep blue (basophilic) cytoplasmic granules.	Allergic reactions; release inflammatory mediators.
Lymphocytes	20-25% of all WBCs.	8-10 µm in diameter; bilobed nucleus; deep blue (basophilic) cytoplasmic granules.	Inmume reactions; antigen-antibody reactions.
Monocytes	3-8% of all WBCs.	12-20 µm; kidney shaped nucles.	Phagocytosis.
Platelets	1.5 lacs to 4 lacs / ml.	2-4 µm diameter; non-nucleated. Lifespan – 5-9 days.	Haemostasis; forms platelet plug.

HAEMOSTASIS

It is prevention of blood loss wherever a vessel is severed or ruptured. Haemostasis is achieved by several mechanisms like vascular spasm, blood clot formation, fibrinous tissue growth, platelet plug formation.

Mechanism of haemostasis :

Severed vessels
↓
Constriction of vessel
↓
Platelets agglutination
↓
Formation of fibrin clot
↓
Appearance of fibrin
↓
Clot retraction

Vascular constriction

Immediately after a blood vessel is cut or ruptured there occurs vasoconstriction of that vessel which reduces blood flow. This vasoconstriction occurs due to nervous reflexes, local myogenic spasm, local humoral factors etc.

Platelet plug formation

Injury to blood vessel exposes underlying collagen and attracts platelets leading to temporary haemostatic plug formation, which is converted to definitive haemostatic plug after the action of fibrin upon temporary haemostatic plug.

Blood coagulation

The clot begins to develop 15 to 20 seconds after the injury or may take 2-3 minutes. Various clotting factors are involved in the blood coagulation. The list of these clotting factors is given in the following table :

Clotting factor	International synonyms
Fibrinogen	Factor-I
Prothrombin	Factor-II
Thromboplastin	Factor-III
Calcium	Factor-IV
Labile factor	Factor-V
SPCA (Serum Prothrombin Conversion Acceletor)	Factor-VI

Anti hemophilic factor	Factor-VIII
Plasma thromboplastin component (Christmas factor)	Factor-IX
Stuart Factor	Factor-X
Plasma thromboplastin antecedent	Factor-XI
Hageman factor (glass factor)	Factor-XII
Fibrin stablizing factor	Factor-XIII
Prekallikerien	Fletcher factor
Platelets	—

Mechanism of blood coagulation : In response to severed vessels a number of chemical reactions occur in the blood involving more than a dozen of blood coagulation factors, leading to formation of prothrombin activator which catalyzes prothrombin to thrombin. This thrombin then converts fibrinogen to fibrin fibres, that meshes platelets, blood cells and plasma leading to formation of blood clot.

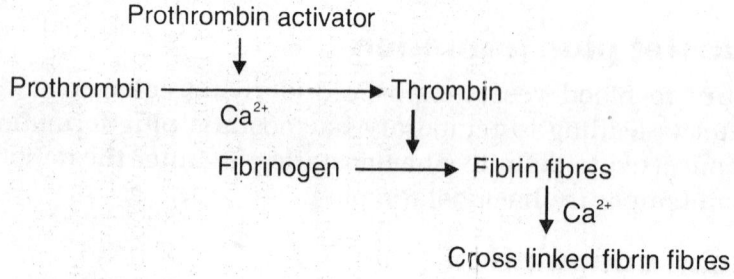

Blood coagulation involves extrinsic and intrinsic systems.

Extrinsic system : It is activated when injury occurs to blood vessel wall. This causes release of tissue factor which in turn activate factor VII and factor X.

Intrinsic system : Intrinsic system is activated when blood is exposed to collegen fibres underlying the endothelium in blood vessels. This activates factors XII which is turn activates factor XI, factor IX, subsequently factor X; finally producing prothrombin activator which forms thrombin as shown in the following flow chart.

Both the extrinsic and intrinsic systems complement each other.

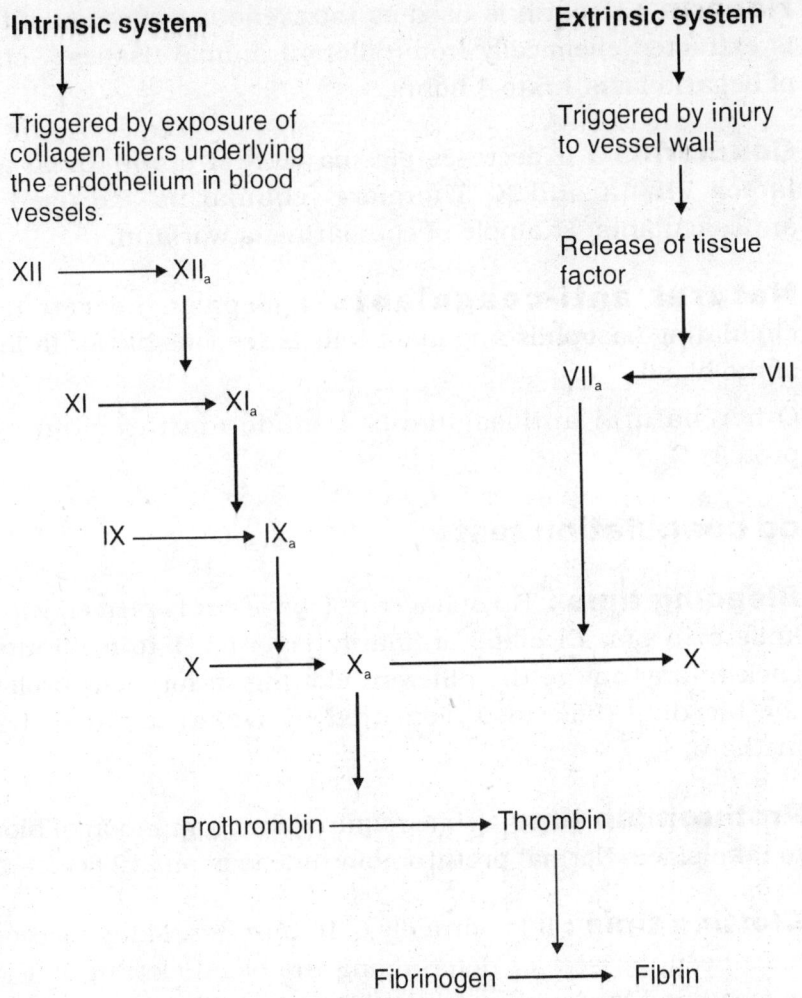

Fig. 6.3 The intrinsic and extrinsic pathways of coagulation.

Plasmin : The plasma proteins contain a globulin known as plasminogen which when activated becomes plasmin.

Plasmin is a proteolytic enzyme that digests fibrin fibres as well as other protein coagulauts. Therefore, plasmin leads to destruction of clotting factors and finally causing lysis of blood clot and hypocoagulability of the blood.

Anti coagulants

Various anti coagulants have been developed. Some of the anticoagulants are natural like Heparin, Protein-C. Some are synthetic like Vit.-K, analogies, Arvin.

Clinical uses of anticoagulents :

Heparin : Heparin is used as intravenous anticoagulant. It is extracted chemically from different animal tissues. Action of heparin lasts 1.5 to 4 hours.

Coumarins : It decreses plasma level of prothrombin and factor VII, IX and X. Therefore, coumarins are used as anticoagulants. Example of coumarins is warfarin.

Natural anti-coagulants : Heparin secreted by circulating basophils and mast cells is responsible for fluidity of the blood.

Other natural anticoagulants include antithrombin and protein-C.

Blood coagulation tests

Bleeding time : Tip of finger or lobe of ear is pierced with a knife or a pin. Bleeding ordinarily lasts for 1 to 6 minutes. Lack of any one of the different clotting factors can prolong the bleeding time; also measured by Duke's method, Ivy's method.

Prothrombin time : Time required for coagulation of blood to take place. Normal prothrombin time is about 12 sec.

Clotting time : It is normally 6-10 minutes. Many methods have been devised for determining the blood clotting time. It is measured by capillary method, Lee and White method.

BLOOD VOLUME

Blood contains both extracellular fluid (fluid in plasma) and intracellular fluid (the fluid in the red blood cells). All fluids outside the cells are collectively called extracellular fluid. These fluids constitute about 20% of body weight. Two largest compartments of extracellular fluid are the interstitial fluid and the plasma. The average blood volume of adults is about 7% of body weight or around 5 liters with pH of 7.4 ± 0.05, i.e. alkaline and viscosity 4-5 times of water. Forty percent is red blood cells and 60% of blood is plasma.

Major cations and anions of E.C.F. and Intracellular fluids:

1. Na^+, Cl^-, HCO_3^- (mainly extracellular)
2. K^+, Mg^{2+}, Cu^{2+}, PO_4^{3-}, Proteins (mainly intracellular)

Normal values for the cellular elements in human blood

	Cells/mm³	Normal range	% of total white cells
Total W.B.C.	9000	4000-11000	—
Granulocytes			
Neutrophils	5400	3000-6000	50-70
Eosinophils	280	150-300	1-5
Basophils	35	0-100	0.4
Lymphocytes	2750	1500-4000	20-40
Monocytes	540	300-600	2-8
Erythrocytes			
♀	4.8×10^6	$3.8 - 5.8 \times 10^6$	—
♂	5.4×10^6	$4.5 - 6.5 \times 10^6$	—
Platelets	300000	1.5 - 4 Lacs/mm³	—

R.B.C. INDICES

R.B.C. indices are used to classify types of anaemias (laboratory classification). The numerical values are calculated from the total number of R.B.Cs, Hb content and the haematocrit values.

MCV (Mean Corpuscular Volume)

It is volume of a single RBC expressed in micrometers³

$$MCV = \frac{\text{Packed cell vol}^m (\%) \times 10}{\text{R.B.C. count (in million/mm}^3 \text{ of blood)}} \; f^3$$

(normal 77-95 µm³)

MCH (Mean Corpuscular Haemoglobin)

Average amount of haemoglobin in a single RBC expressed in picograms.

$$MCH = \frac{\text{Hb (gm\%)} \times 10}{\text{R.B.C. count (in million / mm}^3 \text{ of blood)}} \; Pg$$

(normal 27-32 pg)

MCHC (Mean Corpuscular Haemoglobin Concentration)

It is the amount of haemoglobin expressed as percentage of volume of RBC.

$$MCHC = \frac{Hb\ (gm\%) \times 100}{PCV\ (\%)}$$

(normal value 32-38 %)

Colour Index

It is ratio of two ratios and is interpreted as :

$$CI = \frac{Hb\ (as\ \%\ of\ normal)}{R.B.C.\ count\ (as\ \%\ of\ normal)}$$

(range 0.85-1.15)

Applied physiology

Normochromic – If MCHC is within normal range.

Hypochromic – If MCHC is less than the normal range.

Normocytes – R.B.Cs with normal values of MCV.

Microcytes – R.B.Cs with less than normal size.

Macrocytes – R.B.Cs with more than normal size.

What is meant by osmotic fragility of R.B.Cs – It is defined as the ease with which R.B.Cs are broken down in hypotonic solution.

Normal range 0.47% of Nacl to 0.34% of Nacl solution.

PLASMA PROTEINS

Plasma proteins are derived from mesenchymal cells in embryo. In adults from liver mainly.

		Normal range
Plasma proteins	—	6.4 – 8.3 gm%
Albumin	—	3 – 5 gm%
Globulin	—	2 – 3 gm%
A : G ratio	—	1.7 : 1

Types of plasma proteins :
1. Pre-albumin
2. Albumin
3. Globulin
4. Fibrinogen
5. Prothrombin

The major types of plasma protein present in plasma are albumin, globulin and fibrinogen.

The principle function of albumin is to provide colloid osmotic pressure in the plasma which provide prevention of plasma loss from the capillaries.

The globulin has a number of enzymatic reactions in the plasma. They are responsible for both the natural and the acquired immunity that a person has against invading organisms.

The fibrinogen and prothrombin help in coagulation of the blood.

The plasma proteins help in maintaing the acid-base balance in the body. They are amphoteric in nature, therefore, behave as acids or bases depending upon the conditions.

The plasma proteins are also used as a source of amino-acids for the tissues; there exists a reversible equilibrium between plasma proteins and the tissue proteins.

The plasma proteins are also a source of energy.

Various substances like hormones and drugs are carried in blood by binding to various plamsa proteins that serve as transport proteins.

The various plasma proteins maintain the viscosity of the blood and arterial blood pressure (systematic).

Globulin combine with pigment haem to from haemoglobin which carries oxygen in red blood cells.

HAEMOGLOBIN

It is the oxygen carrying pigment of the red blood cells.

Haem is an iron containing porphyrin. *Globin* is a protein built from four polypeptides chains — two α and two β. Hence, the normal adult haemoglobin is written as HbA ($\alpha_2\beta_2$). Each polypeptide chain is associated with 1 haem group. Therefore, each molecule of Haemoglobin has 4 haem groups which can carry 4 molecules of oxygen. Oxygen - Haemoglobin dissociation curve is sigmoidal in shape. 2-3 DPG, and product of glucose metatolism redcues the affinity of Haemoglobin for oxygen which results in release of oxygen to tissues. At birth the haemoglobin is 23 gm% but in adults haemoglobin is 14-18 gm% in males and 12-15 gm% in females.

The haemoglobin has major role in transport of oxygen from lungs to the tissues and transport of Co_2 from the tissues to the lungs (1 gm% of Haemoglobin can carry 1.34 ml of oxygen). It is also a buffering protein of plasma.

Haemoglobin is split of into Globin and Heam by the tissue-macrophages. The haem is brocken into Fe^{2+} and biliverdin. biliverdin is reduced to Bilirubin. Fe^{2+} is redused or combined with apoferritin to form ferritin. Bilirubin is taken up by liver for conjugation and then excreted in bile.

Other varieties of Haemoglobin include :

1. *Foetal Haemoglobin* – In it the 2 β chains are replaced by 2 γ chains (HbF – $\alpha_2 \gamma_2$). It has greater affinity for oxygen than adult Haemoglobin.
2. *HbS* – In it the β chains contain a valine residue at position 6 in place of a glutamic acid residue present normally. HbS easily precipitates into crystals and causes RBCs to become sickle shaped. RBCs become fragile. The resulting anemia is called *sickle cell anemia.*
3. *Thalassemia* – It is persistence of foetal haemoglobin beyond the age of 4-6 month after birth. It is due to deficient or reduced production of α or β chains.

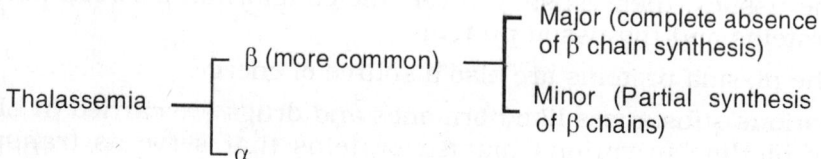

BLOOD GROUPS

Blood grouping is based on the presence or absence of specific antigens on the surface of RBCs.

Chief blood groups are :
1. ABO blood groups
2. Rh blood groups
3. M and N blood groups

ABO blood groups

Two antigens – Type-A and Type-B occur on the surface of the red blood cells in a large proportion of human beings. Relative frequency of different blood types is as following:

    A   41%
    B   9%
    AB   3%
    O   47%

Blood group system (ABO)

Blood group	Genotype	Antigens present on RBC	Antibodies present in plasma
O	OO	None	Anti-A & Anti-B
A	AA, AO	A	Anti-B
B	BB, BO	B	Anti-A
AB	AB	A & B	None

Genetic determination of these agglutinogens (the blood group specific antigens) is by two genes.

Landsteiner's Law : If an antigen is present in the R.B.Cs of an individual the corresponding antibody must be absent from the plasma or if the agglutinogen is absent in the individual's R.B.Cs the corresponding antibody must be present in the plasma.

Rh blood groups

Here the blood group depands on presence or absence of Rh Antigen on RBCs. In Rh–ve persons RBCs lack the D-antigen but their plasma does not contain any anti-D antibody. Rh blood groups are of two types — Rh+ve and Rh –ve. There are six common types of Rh Factors. These are C, D, E, c, d, e.

The type-D is widely prevalent in the population. In Rh system, Rh antibodies are of the IgG type and can cross the placenta. Antigen - antibody reaction occurs best at the body temperature.

When Rhesus monkey R.B.Cs are injected into rabbits, the rabbits responds by forming antibodies which agglutinate Rhesus R.B.Cs.

Though Rh -ve individuals have no naturally occuring antibody against Rh +ve cells but upon antigenic stimulation they produce antibodies against Rh +ve cells.

Erythroblastosis foetalis : In this condition red blood cells of the Rh +ve foetus are attacked by anti-Rh antibodies from Rh –ve mother who has been previously sensitised to Rh antigen by mismatched blood transfusion or as a result of previous pregnancy bearing Rh +ve baby.

M and N blood groups

M and N factors depend upon two minor genes.

Uses of blood grouping

1. To check Rh incompatibility in pregnancy.
2. Before blood transfusion, otherwise haemolysis may occur.
3. Medicolegal value.
4. Paternity disputes.

JAUNDICE

Yellow discolouration of the skin, conjunctiva and mucous membranes due to excessive bilirubin in the tissue fluids and plasma is known as jaundice.

Normal plasma bilirubin

Total — 0.2 – 1.2 mg%.
Direct — 0.1 – 0.4 mg%.
Indirect — 0.2 – 0.8 mg%.

Bilirubin is a product of Haem metabolism. It exists in 2 forms:
1. Direct or conjugated bilirubin — It is water soluble form and cannot cross blood brain barrier.
2. Indirect or unconjugated bilirubin — It is not water soluble and can cross blood brain barrier.

In adults jaundice becomes clinically apparent when bilirubin levels exceed 2 mg%.

Whereas in infants clinical jaundice appears above 5 mg% level.

Causes

1. Excessive breakdown of red blood cells which is called haemolytic jaundice.
2. Obstructive jaundice due to obstruction of bile ducts by stones, carcinoma, etc.
3. Hepatic jaundice is due to damage to the liver; the cause can be infective or toxic.

Synonyms

Pre-hepatic jaundice – Haemolytic jaundice.
Post-hepatic jaundice – Obstructive jaundice.
Hepatic jaundice – Hepato cellular jaundice.

Differences between pre-hepatic, hepatic and post-hepatic jaundice

		Pre-hepatic	**Hepatic**	**Post-hepatic**
1.	Cause	Excessive haemolysis.	Damage to liver. Decreased conjugation. Decreased excretion into bile.	Obstruction of bill ducts.
2.	Type of Bilirubin elevated	Indirect.	Indirect and direct.	Direct.
3.	Urine urobilinogen	Increased.	Decreased.	Absent.
4.	Urine bilirubin	Absent.	Present.	Present.
5.	Faecal stercobilinogen	Increased.	Decreased.	Absent.
6.	Faecal fat	Normal.	Increased[+].	Increased[++].
7.	Liver function tests	Normal.	Impaired.	Normal or slightly impaired.

Physiological jaundice

New born infants develop jaundice due to elevated levels of unconjugated bilirubin during the first week.

Factors responsible for physiological jaundice are :
1. Lifespan of RBCs in newborns is reduced – about 90 days (normal 120 days).
2. Hepatic immaturity – less hepatic conjugation.
3. Increased euterohepaptic circulation in newborns.

GOOD ADVICE IS HARD TO GIVE, BUT EVEN HARDER TO FOLLOW.

7
THE RETICULOENDOTHELIAL SYSTEM

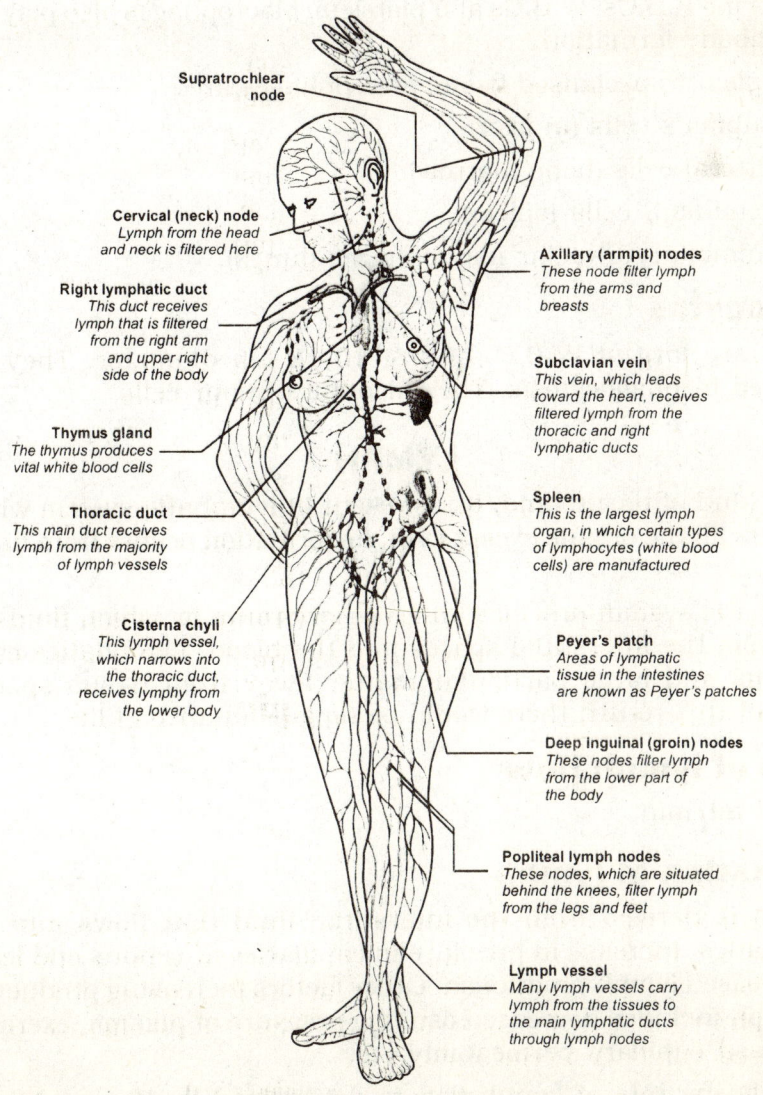

Fig. 7.1 The lymphatic system.

RETICULOENDOTHELIAL SYSTEM

It is the combination of macrophages, monocytes and a few specialized endothelial cells in the bone marrow, spleen and lymph nodes.

Sites of lymphoid tissues are bone marrow, Peyer's patches, spleen, lymph nodes, tonsils, appendix and thymus.

Macrophages

These are specialised phagocytic cells in different parts of body. They are involved in ingestion of bacteria and thus act as a defence line against invasion of bacteria. They are also involved in destroying R.B.Cs, W.B.Cs and platelets. Macrophages also play role in antibody formation.

Examples f specialised tissue macrophages are :

1. Kupffer's cells (in liver).
2. Littoral cells (bone marrow).
3. Reticulam cells (spleen).
4. Pulmonary alveolar macrophages (lungs).

Monocytes

These are largest W.B.C. of size 10-18 μm diameter. They are involved in phagocytosis. They also kill tumour cells.

LYMPH

It is a kind of tissue fluid. It is present in lymphatic system which exists in all the organs except CNS. Its formation occurs from tissue fluids.

Lymphatic system provides an accessory route by which fluid can flow from the interstitial spaces into the blood. Lymphatics carry proteins and large particular matter away from tissue spaces. Without this return there would be no sustainance of life.

Rate of lymph flow

0.5 – 1 ml/min.

Formation of lymph

Lymph is derived from the interstitial fluid that flows into the lymphatics. Increase in pressure in capillaries at venous end leads to increased lymph production. Other factors increasing production of lymph includes decreased osmotic pressure of plasma, exercise, increased capillary permeability etc.

Roughly the rate of lymph flow is determined by the product of interstitial fluid pressure times the activity of the lymphatic pump.

Functions of lymph

1. Protein transportation.
2. Antibiotic transport.
3. Blood cells (R.B.C., W.B.C.) transport.
4. Protein return to vascular system from intenstitial fluid.
5. Large particulate matter transport.
6. Transport of certain enzymes.
7. Transporting the absorbed fatty acids in intestine to the blood vessels.

SPLEEN

Spleen is non-essential part of human body. Its main function is R.B.C. formation. It acts as a R.B.C. reservoir; spleen also forms lymphocytes and plasma cells and it has participation in defence system of human body.

Adult spleen is the largest collection of lymphoidal tissue in the body. It is around 12 cm in length, 7 cm wide and 2.5 cm thick. Its weight is around 150 grams.

Spleen in positioned in the left of abdomen lying between the fundus of the stomach and diaphragm.

Blood supply

Splenic artery.

Functional aspects of spleen

1. Lymphocyte development – The spleen produces T and B lymphocytes
2. The spleen is a part of reticuloendothelial system. It destroys old and worn out RBCs, WBCs and platelets.
3. Reservoir for blood – It releases blood on demand. This is controlled by sympathetic nervous system and helps to maintain the composition of body fluids.
4. Participates in defence against bateria and parasites by phagocytosis and antibody formation.

LYMPH NODES

Lymph nodes are oval shaped masses with a cortex, paracortex and medulla.

Cortex contains B lymphocytes. Paracortex contains T lymphocytes and medulla contains both B and T lymphocytes.

Lymphocytes and antigens enter into the node through the afferent lymphatics. The lymph drains into the node through afferent lymphatics.

The lymph drains through the node and passes out of the medulla of the node through efferent lymphatic vessels.

EDEMA

Edema refers to the presence of excess fluid in the body tissues. Edema can be intracellular edema or extracellular edema or combined edema.

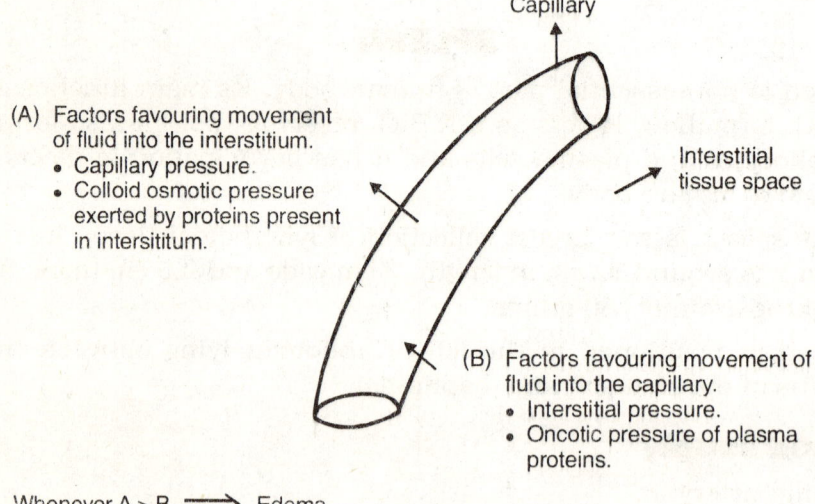

Fig. 7.2 Diagram showing mechanism of edema.

Under normal conditions about 20 litres of fluid per day pass from circulation into the interstitium. Of this 18 litres is reabsorbed by the circulation, either in the tissues or in the lymph nodes. About 2 liters is returned to the circulation as lymph via thoracic duct.

The direction of fluid movement depends upon the following factors:

1. Capillary pressure
2. Interstitial pressure
3. Oncotic pressure by plasma proteins
4. Colloid osmotic pressure of proteins within the interstitial fluid

Treatment of edema in allopathy is by administration of drugs known as diuretics that promote the excretion of both water and sodium. An increase in water excretion alone is not sufficient to eliminate the accumulated fluid. Action of diuretics is by sodium transport inhibition in the nephron or by modifying the filterate.

8

THE CARDIOVASCULAR SYSTEM

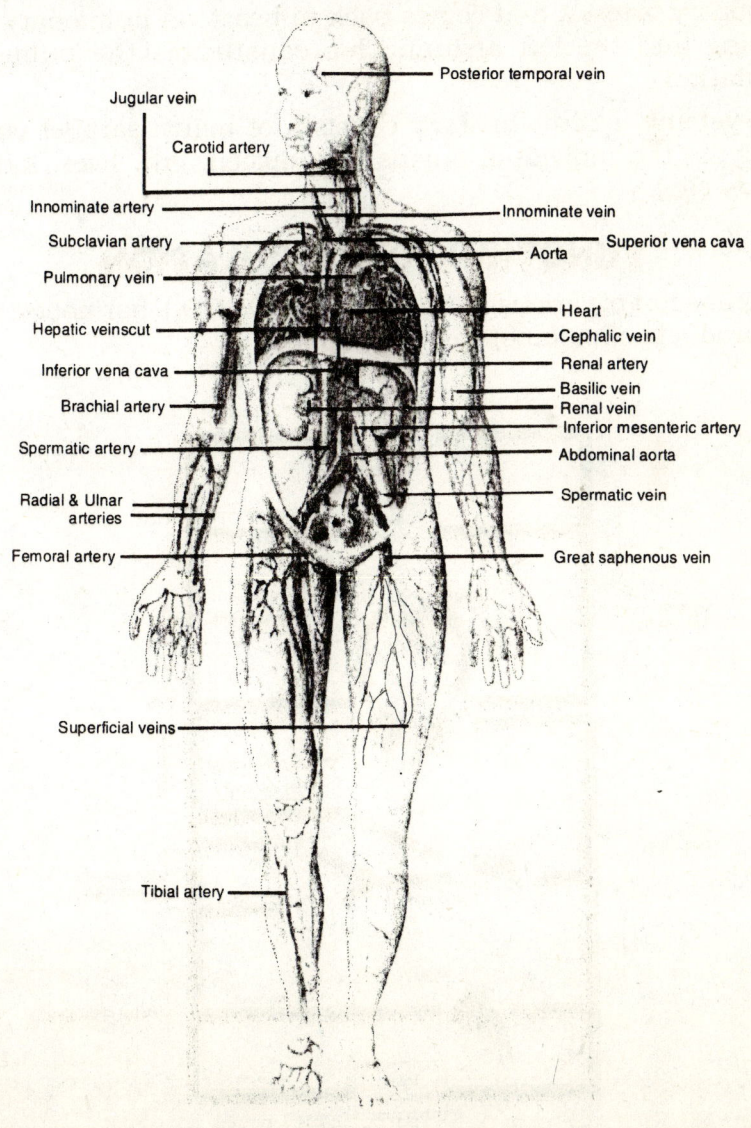

Fig. 8.1 Circulatory system.

ORGANISATION OF CIRCULATION

Circulatory system comprises of a pump (the heart) and blood vessels (arteries, veins, capillaries).

Circulatory system contains two circuits arranged in series – the systemic circulation and the pulmonary circulation.

Blood pumped out from the left ventricle circulates to various body parts and returns back to the heart via superior and inferior vena cava opening in the right atrium. This constitutes the systemic circulation.

Blood pumped out by the right ventricle goes to the lungs via pulmonary arteries and comes back to heart via pulmonary veins opening into the left atrium. This constitutes the pulmonary circulation.

The systemic circuit in itself consists of many parallel circuits supplying the individual organs (e.g. spleen, gut, liver, kidneys, gonads etc.).

FUNCTIONS OF CIRCULATION

1. Transport of various nutrients, gases (O_2, CO_2), hormones, waste products of metabolism etc.

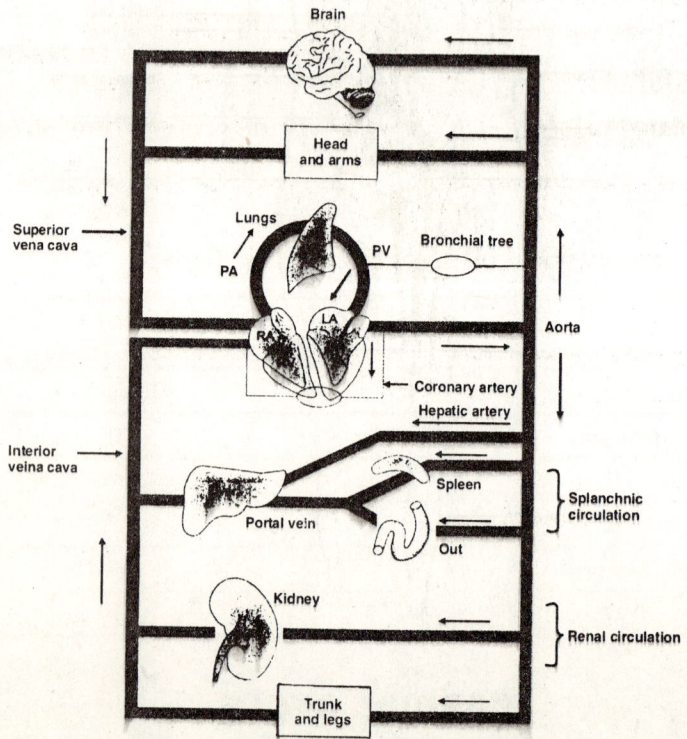

Fig. 8.2 Components of circulatory system.

2. Regulates the composition of extracellular fluid.
3. Circulation plays important role in regulating various physiological functions (e.g. hormonal control, defense against infection, regulation of body temperature).

CARDIAC MUSCLE

1. Made up of many individual cells known as cardiac myocytes linked together via intercalated disks.
2. Have a single nucleus.
3. Striate appearance is due to orderly array of sarcomere.
4. Principle contractile proteins are —
   (a) Actin
   (b) Myosin

Electrical Properties

1. **Excitability** — Cardiac muscle forms a wave of depolarisation (action potential) in response to a stimulus.
2. **Autorhythmicity** — It is the property by virtue of which some specialised cells of the myocardium known as the pacemakers (e.g. SA node, AV node) are capable of generating action potentials on their own without any external stimulation.
3. **Conductivity** — It is property of propagation of cardiac impulse. The speed of propogation of cardiac impulse varies in different parts.

Speed of conduction in different cardiac tissue

Tissue	Speed of conduction (m/s)
SA node	0.05
Atrial pathways	1
AV node	0.05
Bundle of His	1
Purkinje system	4
Ventricular muscles	1

CARDIAC CYCLE

It refers to the cyclical changes occuring in the heart (contraction and relaxation) between two consecutive beats.

Duration

0.8 second (total).

Events

In each cardiac cycle there are 4 main events :
1. Atrial systole – 0.1 sec.
2. Ventricular systole – 0.3 sec.
3. Ventricular diastole – 0.5 sec.
4. Atrial diastole – 0.7 sec.

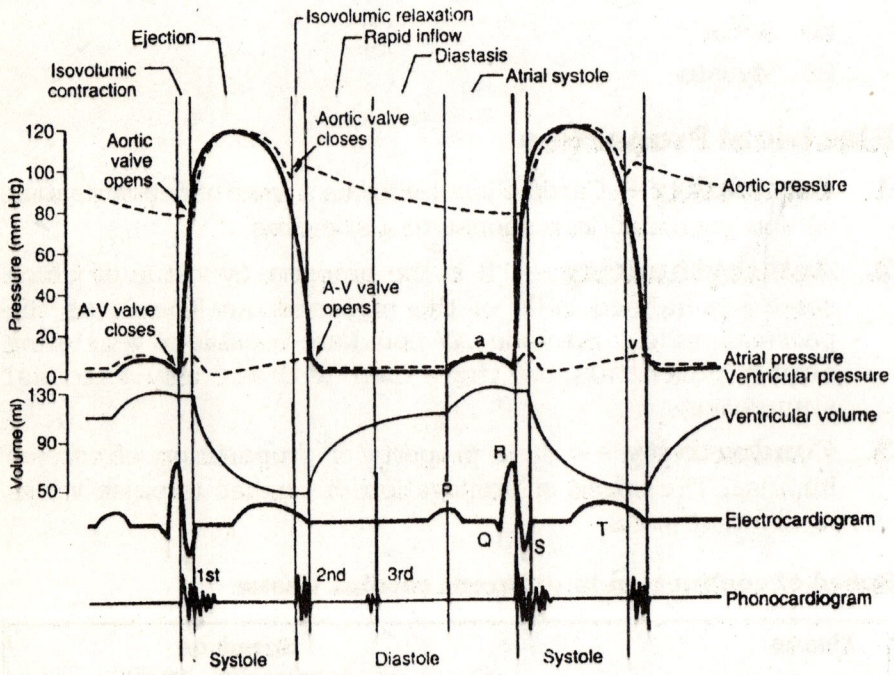

Fig. 8.3 Various events in cardiac cycle.

Since SA node is located in right atnium, therefore, atrial systole is the first phase of cardiac cycle.

It lasts for 0.1 sec. and is followed by atrial diastole lasting 0.7 sec.

At the end of atrial systole ventricular systole starts which lasts for 0.3 sec. Ventricular systole is followed by ventricular diastole lasting 0.5 sec.

The chambers of heart relax and fill with blood during diastole and contract to eject blood during systole.

The total amount of blood filling the ventricles at the end of diastable is called the end diastolic volume. About 2/3rd of this is expelled during systole (about 70 ml) – this is called the stroke volume.

[Note – Depolarisation causes contraction and repolarisation causes relaxation of cardiac muscle fibers. Hence, during systole the cardiac muscle is depolarised and during diastole cardiac muscle undergoes repolarisation].

HEART SOUNDS

They can be heard by auscultation of chest wall with a stethoscope.

Four Hearts Sounds — 2 audible / 2 inaudible

Loud S$_1$

1. Mitral stenosis.
2. Tricuspid stenosis.
3. Thyrotoxicosis.
4. Anemia.

Loud S$_2$

1. Pulmonary hypertension.
2. Systemic hypertension.

First (HS$_1$)

1. Low pitch.
2. Due to AV valve closure
3. Duration – 0.05 sec.

Second (HS$_2$)

1. High pitch
2. Due to semilunar valve closure
3. Duration – 0.025 sec.

Third (HS$_3$)

1. Heard during ventricular diastole due to vibration of cardiac walls.

Fourth (HS$_4$)

1. In atrial systole
2. Normally inaudible

Heart sounds can be heard better over some areas of chest they include :

Area	Site
1. Mitral area	5th intercoastal space (left side) just inner to the midclavicular line.
2. Tricuspid area	Lower end of sterum.
3. Aortic area	2nd right intercoastal space.
4. Pulmonary area	2nd left intercoastal space.

WHAT IS APEX BEAT

It is the lowermost and outermost point of definite cardiac pulsation. It is normally present at 1 cm internal to the mid-clavicular line in the left 5th intercoastal space.

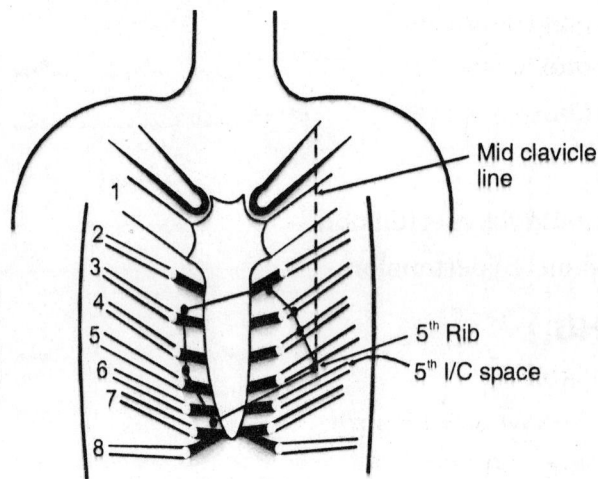

Fig. 8.4 The apex beat.

Apex beat may not be visible in case of :
1. Pericardial effusion.
2. Emphysema.
3. Thick chest wall.
4. Obesity.

Cause

Ventricles contract
↓
Base is pulled downwards and heart rotated to right
↓↓↓

Apex being pushed towards the chest wall
↓
Palpation of beat

ECG

Electrocardiogram is a recording of the electrical activity of the heart during the cardiac cycle, recorded from the body surface.

How to record ECG?

Place electrodes at different points on the body surface and measure voltage difference between them.

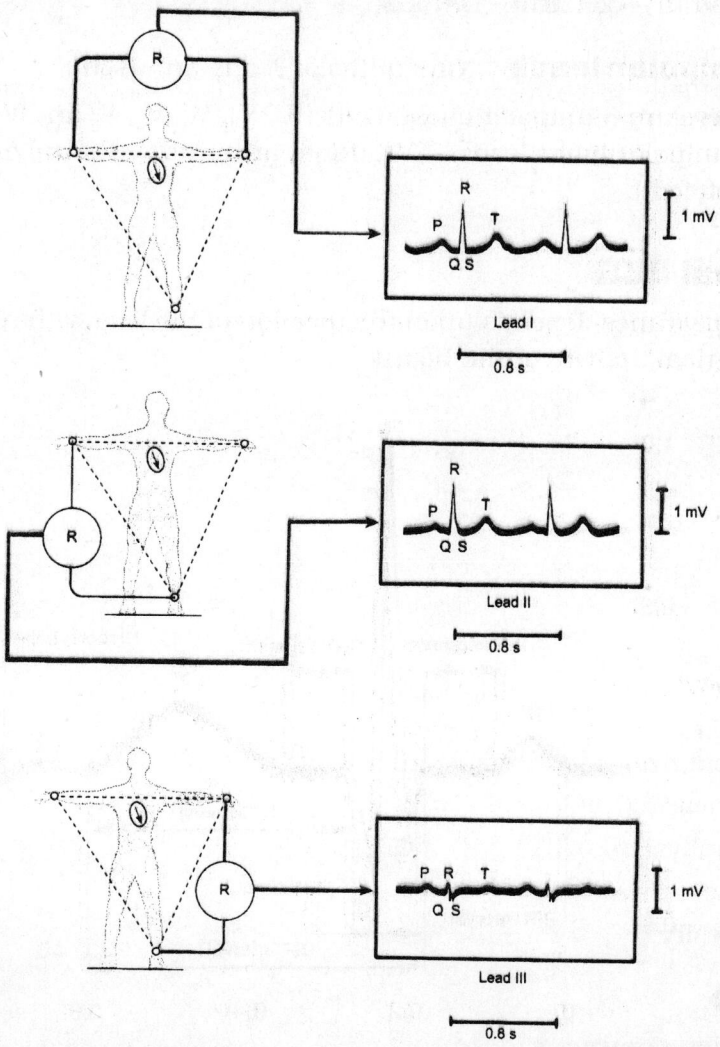

Fig. 8.5 Arrangement of different limb leads used to record ECG.

Unipolar recording : Here an active or exploring electrode is connected to an indifferent electrode at zero potential.

Bipolar recording : Here two active electrodes are used for recording the potential.

Bipolar leads : They include the three standard limb leads. Lead I, II and III are placed on right and left arms and left leg respectively :

Lead I – Right arm – Left arm

Lead II – Right arm – Left leg

Lead III – Left arm – Left leg

Unipolar leads : Nine unipolar leads are used.

There are 6 unipolar chest leads (V_1, V_2, V_3, V_4, V_5 and V_6) and 3 unipolar limbs leads — VR (Right arm), VL (Left arm) and VF (Left foot).

Normal ECG

The appearance depends upon the position of the lead with respect to electrical activity of the heart.

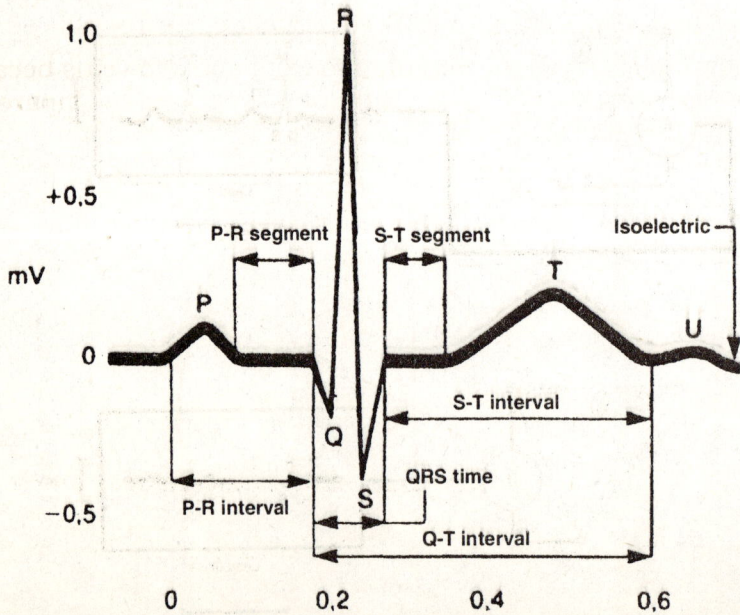

Fig. 8.6 Normal electrocardiogram.

Different waves

Wave	Cause
P wave	— Atrial depolarization.
QRS complex	— Ventricular depolarization.
	Q— Depolarisation of midportion of I.V. septum.
	R— Major portion of both ventricles.
	S— Basal parts of ventricles.
T wave	— Ventricular repolarization.
PR internal	— Delay in transmission through the A.V. node

Use

1. Cardiac abnormalities like arrythmias, ectopic beats, myocardial infarction, heart block, etc. can be detceted.
2. Defect in conducting pathway can be detected.
3. Enlargement of heart can be detected.
4. Detection and localisation of any damage to the heart.

BLOOD DISTRIBUTION AT REST

The data presented in the following diagram shows that small veins and venules contribute to major part of blood distribution system; thus the high proportion of blood is in systemic veins.

Blood flows in the systemic circulation from aorta to veins because of higher pressure in the aorta and other arteries as compared to that in the veins.

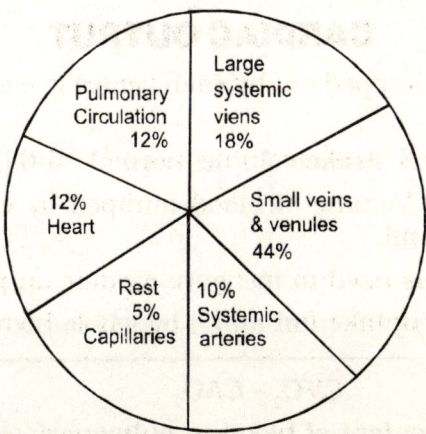

Fig. 8.7 Distribution of blood volume at rest.

The circuation is organised so that the right side of the heart pumps blood through the lungs and left side of heart pumps blood to the rest of the body.

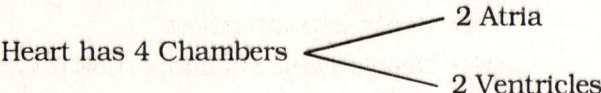

Heart has 4 Chambers — 2 Atria / 2 Ventricles

Mitral and tricuspid valves

1. Mitral valve separates left ventricle from left atrium.
2. Tricuspid valve separates right ventricle from right atrium.
3. These valves prevent reflux of blood into atria when ventricles contract.

Pulmonary and aortic valves

These prevent reflux of blood from pulmonary artery and aorta back into ventricles.

Blood vessels involved

1. Arteries
2. Arterioles
3. Capillaries
4. Venules
5. Veins

Innervation

Smooth muscles of blood vessels are supplied by sympathetic nerve fibres.

CARDIAC OUTPUT

Volume of blood pumped out by each ventricle *each minute is called cardiac output.*

C.O. = Heart rate X stroke volume (normal : 5-6 l/min.).

Stroke volume — Volume of blood pumped by each ventricle *per beat. Normal* – 80 ml.

Fick's principles is used to measure cardiac output :

$$C.O. = \frac{\text{Oxygen uptake (ml min}^{-1}\text{) by whole body}}{CVO_2 - CAO_2}$$

CVO_2 – Oxygen content of blood in pulmonary veins.

CAO_2 – Oxygen content of blood in pulmonary arteries.

Disadvantage of Fick's method :
1. It is an invasive procedure (requires cardiac catheterisation to obtain venous blood sample).
2. Carries risk of infection and trauma.

Changes in either heart rate or stroke volume alters the cardiac output.

Other methods used to measure cardiac output are as follows:
1. Echo-cardiography.
2. Dilution techniques (using dyes or radio-isotopes).

Control of cardiac output
1. Extrinsic autoregulation
2. Intrinsic autoregulation
    (a) Heterometric regulation
    (b) Homometric regulation

Extrinsic autoregulation :
1. It is control of heart rate.
2. Governed by cardiac innervation and cardiovascular centres located in medulla (vasomotor center and cardiac vagal center).

Intrinsic autoregulation :
1. Heterometric regulation.
   Myocardial contractility depends upon resting length of cardiac muscles.
   [**Note** : Force of contraction of heart depand, upon its preload and afterlod.
   Preload refers to the extent to which the myo-cardium is stretched prior to contraction. Preload depands upon :
   (a) End-diastalic volume.
   (b) Venous return to the heart.
   Afterload refers to the resistance against which the ventricles pump out the blood].
2. Homometric regulation
   Myocardial contractility is independent of resting length of cardiac muscle fibres.
   When myocardial contractility is increased it is able to perform more work at the same resting length (i.e. end diastolic volume).

Myocardial contractility is:

Increased by	*Decreased by*
1. Sympathetic stimulation.	1. Para-sympathetic stimulation.
2. Catecholamines.	2. Heart failure.

3. Drugs like
  – Digitalis.
  – Dopamine.
  – Dobutamine.
	3. Myocardial infarction.
	4. Drugs like barbiturates, quinicline.

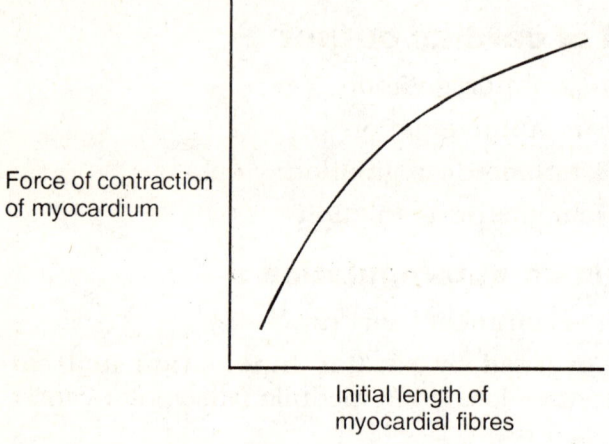

Heterometric regulation of cardiac output.

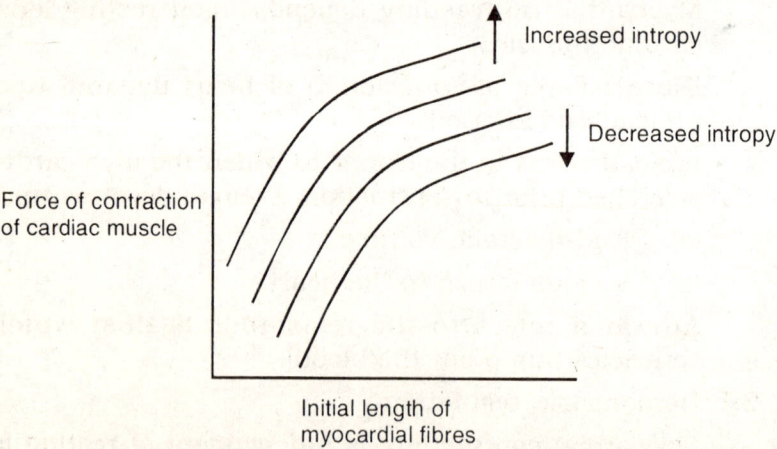

Hemometric regulation of cardiac output.

Fig. 8.8 Intrinsic autoregulation of cardiac output.

Effect of sympathetic and parasympathetic stimulation on cardiac output

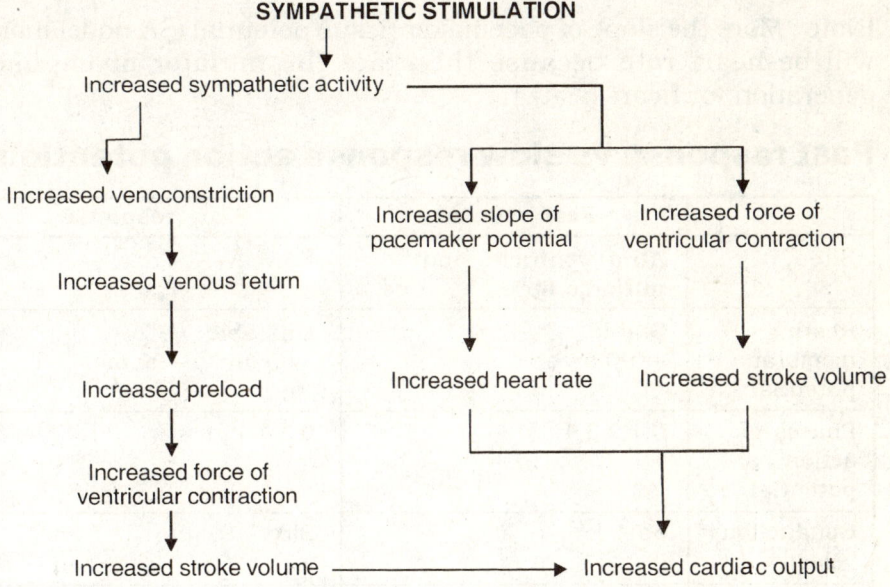

Sympathetic activity causes venoconstriction and increase in slope of pacemaker potential with increased force of ventricular contraction which finally leads to increase in cardiac output as depicted in the above flow chart.

Preload is the amount of blood in the chamber which finally decides the initial length of myocardial fibre and thence force of contraction.

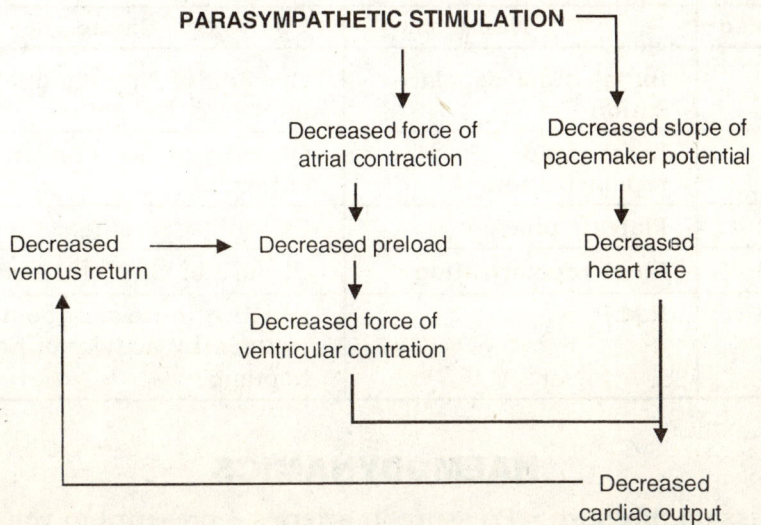

Parasympathetic stimulation leads to decrease in force of atrial contractions and decrease in slope of pacemaker potential which finally leads to decrease in cardiac output as depicted in the above flow chart.

[Note : More the slope of pacemaker tissue potential (SA node) more will be heart rate because these are the initiator of impulse generation for heart beat].

Fast response vs slow response action potentiols

	Fast response	Slow response
Site	Atria, ventricles and purkinje fibres	SAN, AVN
Resting membrane potential	Stable — 90 mv	Unstable – 60 mv to – 90 mv
Phases of action potential	0,1,2,3,4	0,3,4
Conduction velocity	Fast	Slow
Action potential		

Phase	Name	Cause
0	Initial rapid depolarization	Opening of Na+ channel Increased Na+ influx
1	Inital rapid repolarization	Closure of Na+ channel K+ efflux
2	Plateau phase	Ca^{2+} influx K+ efflux
3	Final repolarization	Closure of Ca^{2+} channels
4	R.M.P.	Resting ionic composition restored by activity of Na+ – K+ pump

HAEMODYNAMICS

Perfussion pressure = Pressure in arteries – pressure in veins.

$$\text{Blood flow} = \frac{\text{Perfusion pressure}}{\text{Vascular resistance}}$$

Blood pressure

It is defined as lateral pressure exterted by blood on vessel wall while flowing through it.

Normal — 120/80 mm Hg.

Components of systemic arterial blood pressure :
1. Pulse pressure
2. Mean blood pressure
3. Systolic blood pressure
4. Diastolic blood pressure

Measurement of Blood Pressure by auscultation:
1. A device used for recording blood pressure is known as sphygmomanometer.
2. The cuff is inflatted until the radial pulse can no longer be felt.
3. Korotkoff sounds – Sound pruduced due to turbulent flow in the brachial artery which can be heard during anscultation distal to the cuff when compression is slowly released.
4. Silent gap is sometimes noted in hypertensive patients.

Factors affecting Blood Pressure :

Age : Increase with age.

Body : Obese individuals have high readings.

Climate : Cold → increases

Warm → decreases

Diurnal variation : Afternoon → Peak value

Morning → Lowest

Exercise : Increases with exercise

Gravity : When a subject stands up, pressure is increased in all the viens below the heart and is reduced in all those above the heart as a result of gravity.

(Mnemonics* ABCDEG)

Determinants of arterial B.P. : Main determinants of arterial B.P. are :

1. Cardiac output
2. Peripheral resistance } B.P. = CO x PR

Resistance is determined by the :
1. Caliber of the vessel.
2. Elasticity of vessel wall.
3. Viscosity of blood (determined by haemocrit).
4. Total volume of blood in the circulatory system.

Blood flow in arteries is pulsatile ($\uparrow^{ed}$ during systole and $\downarrow^{ed}$ during diastole).

Systolic pressure – Pressure at the peak of ejection.

Diastolic pressure – Pressure during relaxation.

Veins are capacitance vessels which contain 2/3rd of total blood volume. At heart level veinous pressure is 2 mmHg.

- Resistance offered by capillaries is little, steady.

Determinants – Calibre of the arterioles supplying a particular capillary bed.

Regulation of arterial Blood Pressure :
The various mechanisms for maintining arterial blood pressure are :

1. Nervous regulatory mechanisms — These are rapidly acting B.P. regulatory mechanisms. These act quickly in response to any derangement in blood pressure and prevant B.P. from rising very high or falling very low.

    These mechanisms are :

    (a) Baroreceptor reflexes

    (b) Chemoreceptor reflexes and

    (c) CNS ischaemic response

2. Intrinsic physical regulatory mechnisms — These mechanisms take minutes to few hours to come to play for correcting any derangement in blood pressure.

    These mechanisms are :

    (a) Capillary fluid shift mechanism —

    when B.P. is raised → Increased hydrostatic pressure in capillary bed

    ↓

    Restoration ← Decreased blood   Favours movement
    of B.P.   volume   ← of fluid out of the
                                        capillaries into the
                                        interstititum

    (b) Stress relaxation and reverse stress relaxation mechanisms.

3. Autoregulation of blood pressure by kidneys — It is a long term B.P. regulatory mechanism. It takes few days for this mechanism to become fully active.

Various mechanisms by which kidneys regulate B.P. are :

(a) Renal fluid mechanism
(b) Renin – Angiotensin mechanism and
(c) Aldosterone mechanism

PECULIARITES OF CEREBRAL CIRCULATION

1. Adult brain is about 1400 grams in weight.
2. Brain recieves about 13% of total cardiac output, which is about 750 ml/min.
3. Cerebral oxygen consumption is very high (about 20% of the whole body at rest).
4. Cerebral blood flow is maintained by autoregulation.

    Mechanisms :

    (a) Local metabolite control.
    (b) Basal myogenic tone of blood vessels.
    (c) Cholinergic sympathetic nerves.
5. Anaesthetic agents reduce metabolism and also reduce the cerebral blood flow.
6. Brain tissue is highly sensitive to hypoxia, and hypoxia if prolonged can lead to irreversible neurological deficit.

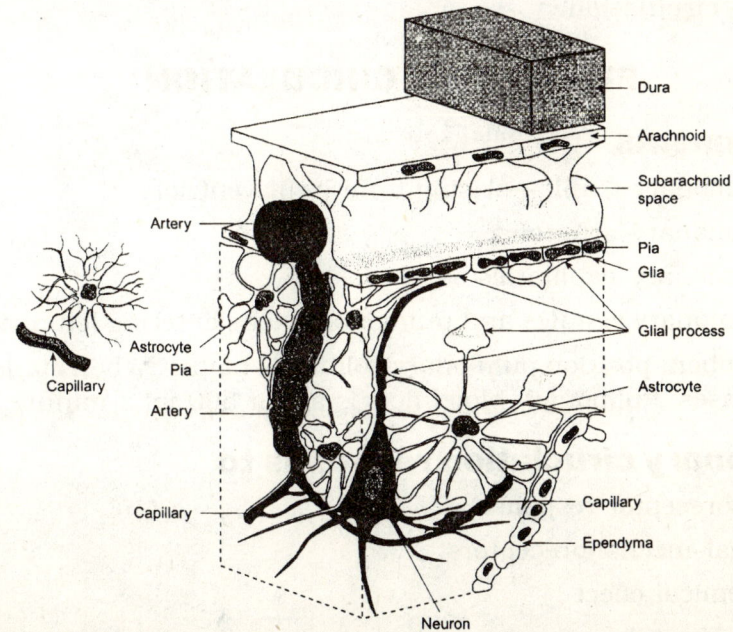

Fig. 8.9 The arrangement of the capillary endothelium and astrocyte end-feet in the cerebral circulation.

Blood brain barrier

It is the barrier that exists between the blood and brain tissue and prevents the entry of various harmful and toxic substances into the brain.

Sites : Choroid plexus; other sites than choroid plexus.

Components of BBB :
1. Tight junctions between endothelial cells in brain capillaries.
2. Brain capillaries are surrounded by foot process of astrocytes.

Permeability :
1. Water, erythromycin, CO_2 and O_2
2. Na^+, K^+, Mg^{2+}

Not permeable : Protein, bile salts and urea.

Functions :
1. Protects cortical neurons from ionic changes.
2. Protection from endogenous and exogenous toxins in the blood.
3. Prevents entry of neurotransmitters into general circulation.

PULMONARY CIRCULATION

Components
1. Pulmonary trunk – arising from right ventricle
2. Pulmonary arterioles
3. Pulmonary capillaries
4. Pulmonary venules and pulmonary veins entering left atrium.

In recumbent position pulmonary volume is higher. When standing it decreases. Pulmonary blood flow is about 500 ml / minute.

Pulmonary ciruclation responds to
1. Baroreceptor response
2. Vagal mechanoreceptors.
3. Chemical effect :
   (a) Hypoxia
   (b) Hypercapnia

SKIN CIRCULATION

1. Its principle role is in thermoregulation achieved by large variations in the blood flow to the skin.
2. On exposure to cold cutaueous blood flow is reduced thus conserving heat.
3. On exposure to heat cutaneous blood flow is increased thus promoting heat loss.
4. Cutaneous circulation is characterised by presence of arterio-venous anastomoses.

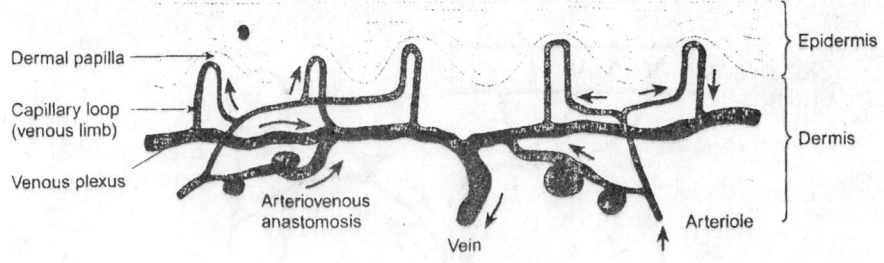

Fig. 8.10 Circulation in skin.

TRIPLE RESPONSE

Normal reaction to injury leads to a three part response:
1. Red reaction
2. Flare
3. Wheal

Red reaction – Reddening at the site of injury.

↓ followed by

Flare – Spreading out of redness.

↓ finally

Wheal – Local diffuse swelling.

Red reaction
Due to dilatation of pre-capillary sphincters in response to release of chemical mediators like – histamine and bradykinin.

Flare
Dilatation of arterioles and precapillary sphincters in the surrounding skin due to *Axon reflex*.

Wheal

1. Increased capillary permeability.
2. Increase in capillary pressure.

Axon reflex

It is local neuronal response.

When a firm stroke is applied across the skin, the afferent impulse are relayed down branches of sensory nerves (dorsal nerve root) to the endings near cutaneous arterioles where it releases a vasodilator substance. It does not involve central nervous system.

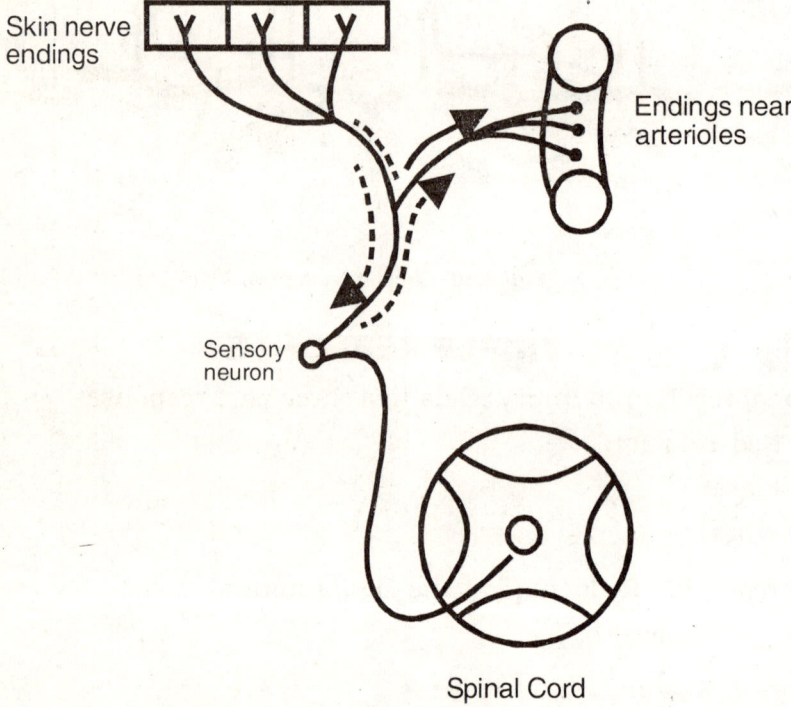

Fig. 8.11 The axon reflex.

CARDIOVASCULAR REGULATION

1. Local autoregulatory mechanisms.
2. Systemic regulatory mechanisms.

Local autoregulatory mechanisms

Auto regulation is the capacity of tissues and organs to maintain their own blood flow.

Resting myogenic tone : Intrinsic capacity to regulate changes in perfusion pressure. It is regulated by sympathetic constrictor nerves.

Factors affecting basal myogenic tone :
1. Local vasodilator metabolites, e.g., hypoxia, hypercapnia, acidemia, lactic acid, increased osmolality.
2. Local vasoconstrictors, e.g., seratonin.

Systemic regulatory mechanisms
1. Neural regulation
2. Chemical regulation

1. Neural regulation :
(a) *Medullary regulation* – It is with the involvement of vasomotor centre and cardiac vagal centre located in medulla.

(b) *Autonomic regulation* – It involves cardiac and peripheral vascular innervation by sympathetic and parasympathatic nerves.

Autonomic regulation :

Cardiac
  (i) Sympathetic ($T_1 - T_5$)
  (ii) Parasympathetic (Vagus)

Peripheral vascular :

  Vasodilators
   (i) Dorsal root vasodilation.
   (ii) ↓^{ed} Sympathetic activity.

  Vasoconstrictions
   (i) ↑^{ed} Sympathetic activity

Medullary regulation : VMC and cardiac vagal centre

  Influenced by :
   (i) Chemoreceptors
   (ii) Baroreceptors

  Cardiovascular regulation helps in :
   (i) Increase in blood supply to active tissues.
   (ii) ↑ or ↓ in heat loss of body helps in thermoregulation.

(iii) Maintainence of blood flow to vital organs in emergencies.

Factors influencing basal myogenic tone :

(a) Local vaso constrictors – cause vasoconstrication of blood vessels.

   (i) ↓ in body temperature

   (ii) 5 HT (serotonin)

(b) Local vasodilators – (cause vasodilatation of blood vessels).

   (i) ↓^{ed} Body pH

   (ii) ↓^{ed} arterial O_2

   (iii) Lactic acid

2. Chemical Regulation :

(a) *Circulating vasoconstrictors*

   (i) Angiotensin II

   (ii) High dose of vasopressin

   (iii) Catecholamines (epinephrine, norepinephrine)

(b) *Circulating vasodilators*

   (i) Bradykinin

   (ii) Kalidin

BARORECEPTORS
(Also known as mechanoreceptors)

These are sensitive to stretch.

Cardiac

Located in the walls of heart.

Arterial

1. Aortic baroreceptors
2. Carotid baroreceptors

Blood pressure is monitored by baroreceptors present in the walls of *aortic arch* and *carotid sinuses*. A rise in blood pressure results in increase in firing of baroreceptor afferents that lead to reflex slowing of heart, peripheral vasodilation and a fall in blood pressure.

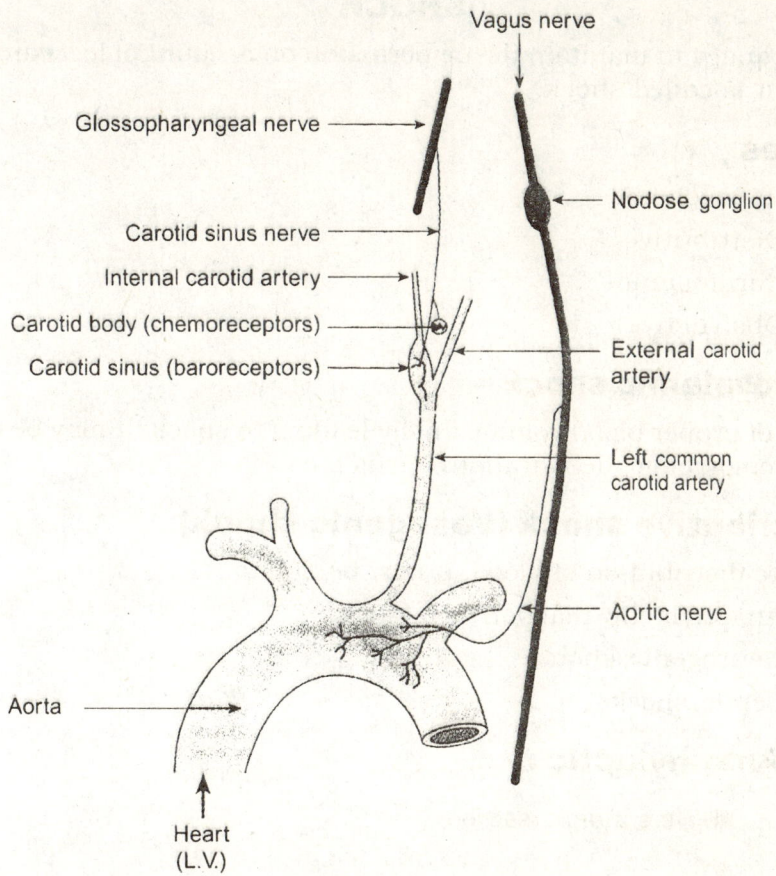

Fig. 8.12 Diagram showing baroreceptors and chemoreceptors.

CHEMORECEPTORS

These detect change in blood chemistry.

Types

Aortic bodies – Located in the aortic arch.

Carotic bodies – Located at the bifurcation of common carotid artery.

These bodies get stimulated by chemical changes in blood such as:
1. Hypoxia
2. Hypercapnia
3. Fall in blood pH.

Afferents from these chemoreceptors relay in *nucleus of tractus solitarius in medulla.*

SHOCK

Inadequacy to maintain tissue perfusion on account of low cardiac output is called shock.

Types

1. Hypovolemic
2. Distributive
3. Cardiogenic
4. Obstructive

Hypovolemic shock

Lack of proper blood volume finally leading to shock. It may be due to haemorrhage, dehydration, burns etc.

Distributive shock (Vasogenic shock)

Due to distribution of blood. It may be due to :

(a) Anaphylactic reaction
(b) Neurogenic shock
(c) Septic shock

Anaphylactic :

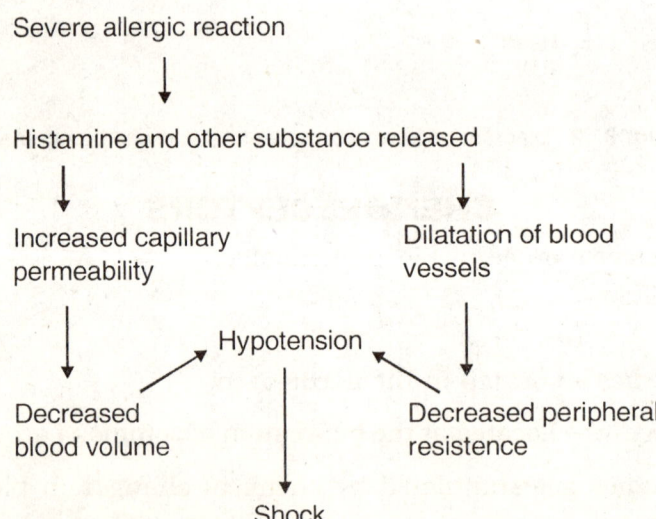

Neurogenic : This occurs due to decrease in cerebral blood flow which may be the result of :

1. Strong emotions such as fear – sympathetic vaso-dilation.
2. Postural hypotension – due to pooling of blood in dependant parts on standing.

Septic shock : Seen in septaecemia due to release of bacterial toxins.

Cardiogenic shock
Due to decreased cardiac output.

Causes :
1. Arrythmia
2. Infarction of cardiac muscle

Obstructive shock
Due to mechanical obstruction to right or left ventricular filling.

Causes :
1. Emboli
2. Cardiac tamponade
3. Tension pneumothorax

Irreversible shock (Refractory shock)
Shock which is not overcomed by compensatory mechanisms or by appropriate treatment.

Signs and symptoms of shock
1. Blood pressure is reduced.
2. Rapid tready pulse.
3. Rapid shallow breathing.
4. Skin is cold, pale and clammy.
5. Altered mental state due to reduced oxygen supply to brain.
6. Urine output is reduced.
7. Acidosis.
8. Intense thirst.
9. Nausea

CARDIAC IMPULSE
It originate from pacemaker tissue of heart.

Pacemaker tissue are certain tissue in the heart, concerned with initiation and propagation of heart beat. This includes :
1. Sino atrial node (SAN)
2. Atrioventricular node (AVN)
3. Bundle of His
4. Purkinje fibres

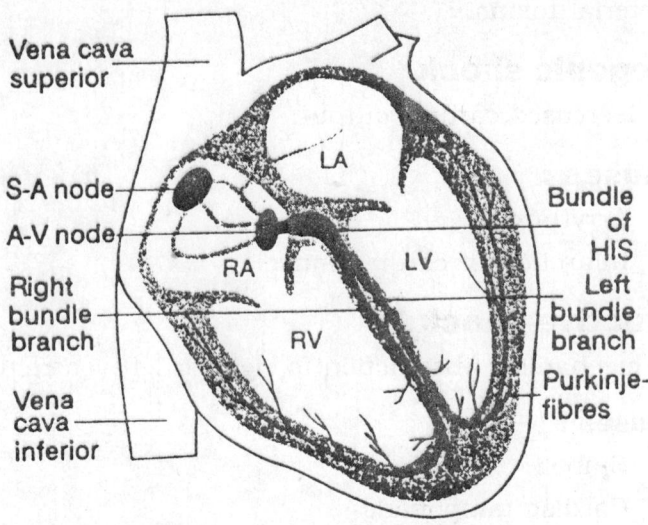

Fig. 8.13 The special conducting system of the heart.

Heart beats spontaneously. It shows an inherent rhythmicity which is independent of any extrinsic nerve supply. Initiation of excitation takes place in specialized group of cells in sino atrial node which lies close to the point of entry of great veins into right atrium. Then a wave of depolarisation is conducted through the myocardium.

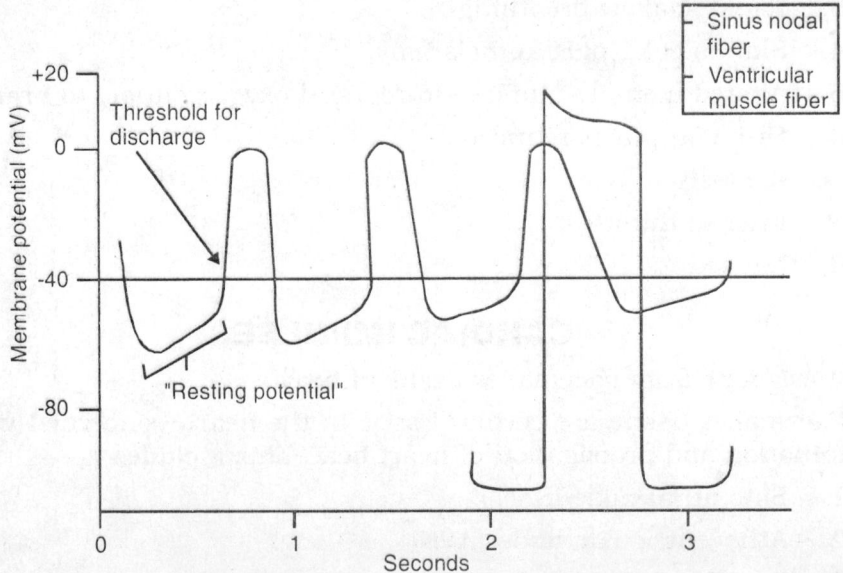

Fig. 8.14 Action potential in myocardial cells.

When threshold is reached in sino atrial node an action potential is triggered to initiate heart beat.

Myocytes of ventricles, artia and conductive system have action potentials with different characteristics.

From the sino atrial node, excitation spreads first across the whole atria. It then passes to venticles via the atrio ventricular (AV) node, which forms the only bridge of conducting tissue between venticles and atria. The conduction through AV node is slow, leading to a delay of 0.1 sec. This ensures that atria have time to contract before the ventricle muscle is excited. Rest of conduction is fast which is mediated by the *Bundle of His*. The Bundle of His divides into the left and right bundle branches supplying the left and right ventricles respectively. This finally terminates in Purkinje fibres in the subendocardium. These fibres in turn spread the excitation to ventricular myocytes. Since the conduction through the Purkinje system is much faster then through the myocardium itself, therefore, all parts of the ventricle are excited at much the same time.

THE VASCULAR SYSTEM

Circulation is achieved because of following types of blood vessels:

1. Distensible vessels
2. Exchange vessels
3. Resistance vessels
4. Capacitance vessels
5. Thoroughfare vessels

Distensible vessles

1. Highly elastic.
2. The stretch produced during cardiac contraction on the walls of the elastic tissues of aorta and its branches comes back to normal original diastolic position.
3. E.g. – aorta.

Exchange vessels

Offer exchange of gases and nutritive substances across them.

They may be :

1. Discontinnous
2. Continuous
3. Fenestrated
4. E.g. – capillaries

Resistance vessels

Offer resistance to blood flow towards the capillaries, e.g. - arterioles.

Capacitance vessels

These vessels change their luminal shape that accommodate larger volume of blood.

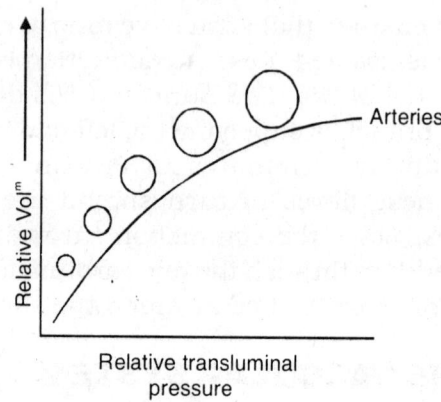

Thoroughfare vessels

These vessels directly connect the arterioles with venules, bypassing the capillaries.

BLOOD FLOW

Blood flow through a vessel can be of two types :
1. Laminar
2. Turbulent flow

Laminar flow	**Turbulent flow**
(i) No noise	Noisy flow
(ii) Blood flows in large number of layers in same direction.	Blood flows in different directions.
(iii) 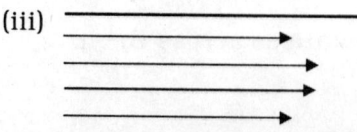	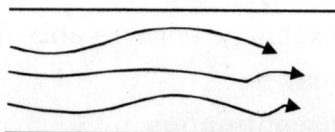
(iv) Present in most parts of vascular system.	Aorta and ventricles mainly.

If the radius of blood vessel is small lesser tension in the walls is necessary to balance the distending pressure.

This is advantage of thin walled and delicate capillaries which makes them less prone to rupture.

CUSHING REACTION

It is a specialized type of response seen in ischaemia of central nervous system, which results from increased pressure of the cerebrospinal fluid around the vault.

The cushing reaction helps to protect the vital centers of the brain from loss of nutrition even if the CSF pressure increases much as to compress the cerebral arteies.

CARDIAC DEPRESSION

When coronary blood flow decreases below that required for adequate nutrition of the myocardium, it weakens the cardiac muscle and finally leads to decrease in cardiac output.

**MOST OF US WILL NEVER DO GREAT THINGS;
BUT WE ALL CAN DO SMALL THINGS IN GREAT WAY.**

9

THE DIGESTIVE SYSTEM

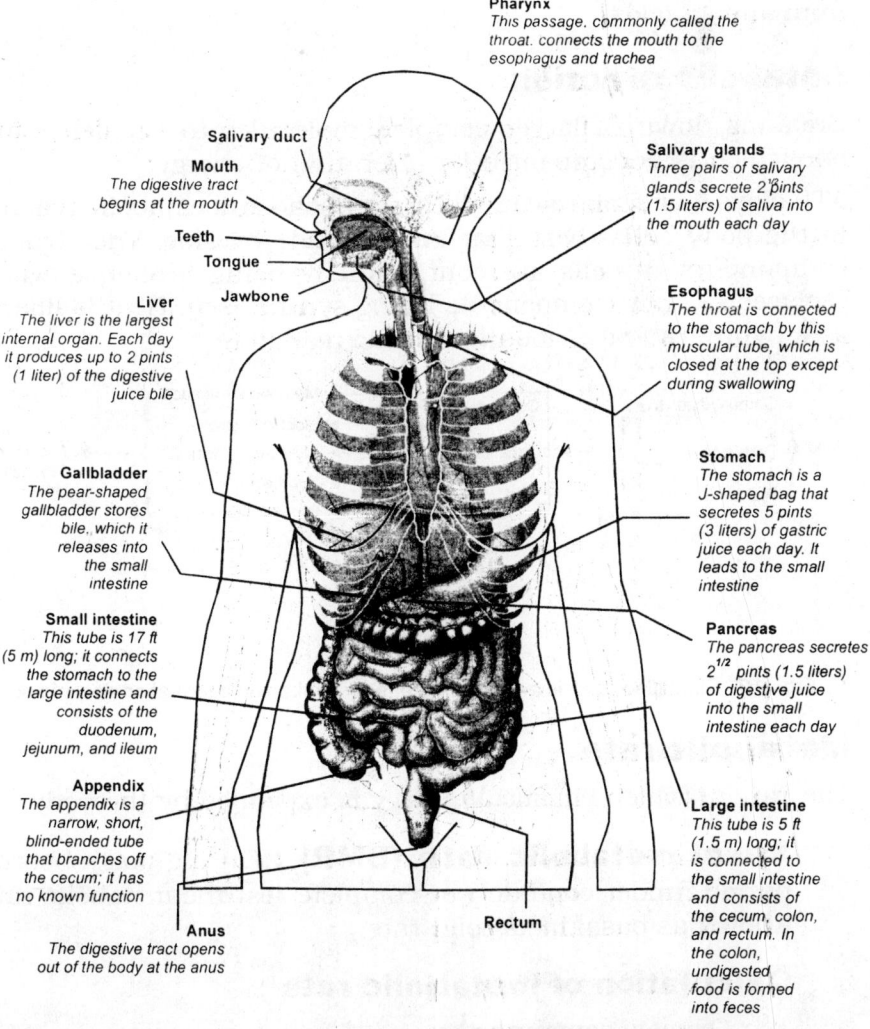

Fig. 9.1 The digestive system.

INTRODUCTION

The vital processes in the body involve a number of chemical reactions. The chemical processes of the body collectively constitute metabolism.

METABOLISM

Metabolism is of two types :
1. Anabolic reaction
2. Catabolic reaction

Anabolic reaction

Synthesis of complex molecules from simpler ones, e.g. – proteins from amino acids.

Catabolic reaction

Breaking down of larger complex molecules to smaller, simpler one which is accompanied by liberation of energy.

ATP plays a crucial role in all the anabolic and catabolic reactions. In the body cells these reactions go side by side. The structural components of cells are continuously being broken down and replaced — new components being synthesised. Heat is liberated as a byproduct of various metabolic reactions.

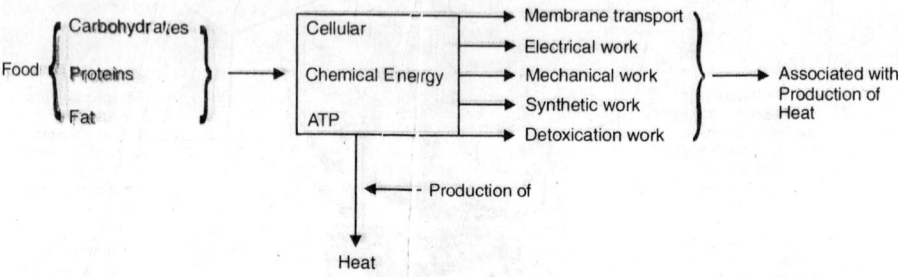

Fig. 19.2 Simplified overview of how the energy intake and information occur in body.

Metabolic rate

The rate at which chemical energy is expended by the body.

Basal metabolic rate (BMR) : During post-absorptive period, under condition of complete rest the metabolic rate is known as basal metabolic rate.

Calculation of metabolic rate :
1. Oxygen consumption
2. Respiratory quotients

3. Any form of exercise, fever, injection of food increases metabolic rate.
4. Malnutrition and sleep decreases metabolic rate.
5. Metabolic rate is also affected by various hormones, e.g., catecholamines and thyroid hormones increase the metabolic rate.

HUMAN BREAST MILK

During gestation, progesteron and oestrogen inhibit the lactogenic action of prolactin but after delivery this inhibitory influence is lost and lactation starts.

Composition of milk changes during the first weeks after parturition.

After delivery during first few days colostrum is secreted. It contains:

High contents of:
1. Proteins
2. Minerals
3. Immunoglobulin

Low contents of:
1. Fats
2. Sugar

The composition of human milk changes gradually over the first week after delivery. By three weeks mature milk is produced. This contains mainly :

High contents of:
1. Proteins
2. Fats
3. Sugar

Low contents of:
1. Minerals
2. Immunoglobulins

Major milk proteins are :
1. Casein
2. α–Lactalbumin
3. Lactoglobulin

Major milk sugar : Lactose.

Composition (approximate) of human breast milk

	Colostrum	Transitional milk	Mature milk
Fat (gl^{-1})	29	34	45
Protein (gl^{-1})	24	15	10
Lactose (gl^{-1})	56	65	70
Caloric value (MJl^{-1})	2.8	3	3

Physiology of milk production and ejection

Production of milk involves interaction of some hormones and reflexes.

These are :

Hormone   **Reflex**

1. Prolactin   —   Prolactin reflex (milk secretion reflex).
2. Oxytocin   —   Oxytocin reflex (milk ejection reflex).

Prolactin reflex : This hormone is produced by anterior pituitary gland.

When the baby sucks at nipples the impulses are carried to the anterior pituitary which in turn releases prolactin hormone.

Prolactin acts on the alveolar cells in the breast, promoting milk secretion.

Oxytocin reflex : This hormone is produced by posterior pituitary gland.

When the baby sucks at the nipple impulses are carried to the posterior pituitary which secretes the oxytocin hormone.

Oxytocin acts on the myoepithelial cells surrounding the alveolar glands in breast. Myoepithelial cells contract and this ejects the milk from the alveolar glands into the lactiferous ducts and sinuses.

DIGESTIVE SYSTEM

Each day an average adult consumes around 1 kg of solid food and 1-2 liters of fluids.

The digestive system breaks down the material into simpler molecules so that it can be used by body for cellular metabolism.

Digestive process includes

Ingestion of food.
↓

Transport of food through the gastrointestinal tract.
↓

Secretion of fluids, salts and digestive enzymes; digestion and absorption of the products of digestion.
↓

Defecation (removal of indigestable remains from the body).

GASTROINTESTINAL TRACT

Parts
1. Oral cavity
2. Pharynx
3. Oesophagus
4. Stomach
5. Small intestine
6. Large intestine
7. Anal canal

Accessory organs
1. Tongue
2. Teeth
3. Salivary glands
4. Exocrine pancreas
5. Liver
6. Gall bladder

General structural features of gut
1. Serosa
2. Longitudinal smooth muscle
3. Circular smooth muscle
4. Submucosa
5. Mucosa

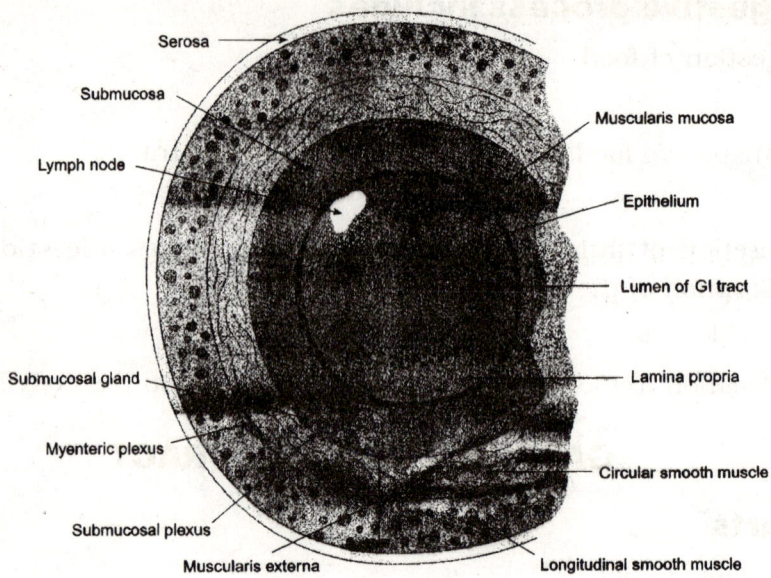

Fig. 9.3 General plan of different layers in the wall of gut.

Contractile activity of smooth muscles promotes mixing and propulsion of food. Contractile activity in the smooth muscle of GI tract is of two types :

1. Segmental involvement
2. Peristaltic contraction

Innervation of gastrointestinal tract

Enteric nervous system is a system of intramural plexuses which mediate a number of intrinsic reflexes that control secretory and contractile activity of the gastrointestinal tract.

Inervation is of 4 types :

Intrinsic :
1. Myenteric plexus
2. Meisner's plexus

Extrinsic :
1. Sympathetic nerves
2. Parasympathetic nerves

Parasympathetic nerves :
1. Vagus
2. Sacral – $S_{2,3,4}$

Sympathetic :
1. $T_6 - T_{12}$
2. $L_1 - L_2$

Hormonal Control

Endocrine and exocrine hormones also play an important role in regulating GI tract activities.

The hormones that regulate GIT :

1. Secretin
2. Gastrin
3. Cholecystokinin (CCK)
4. Gastric inhibitory polypeptide (GIP)
5. Pancreatic polypeptide
6. Motilin
7. Neurotensin

Blood supply

20-30% of cardiac output goes to splanchnic circulation.

Splanchnic circulation : It is combined blood supply to:
1. Stomach and intestine
2. Liver and spleen
3. Pancreas

FUNCTIONS OF ORAL CAVITY

Food intake, chewing and salivary secretion. Food is ingested via mouth. Mixed with saliva and chewed.

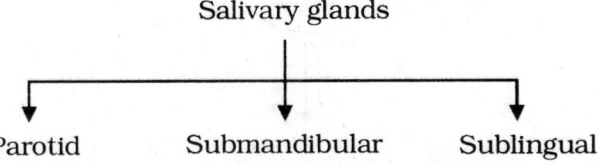

Salivary gland consists of two types of cells :
1. Serous cells
2. Mucous cells

1500 ml of saliva is secreted each day.

Contents of saliva

Mucus – Lubricates the food.

α amylase – Initiates breakdown of carbohydrate.

Lysozymes.

Lipase – Lipolytic enzyme

IgA

Na^+, K^+, Ca^{2+}

HCO_3^-, Cl^-

Urea, creatin

Secreation of saliva

Secreation of saliva is controlled by autonomic nervous system.
1. Parasympathetic nervous system stimulate :
    (a) Abundant Secretion of watery saliva.
    (b) Increased blood flow to salivary gland.
2. Sympathetic nervous system :
    (a) Decreases amylase
    (b) Increases blood flow to gland
    } ⟶ Decreases rate of salivary secretion

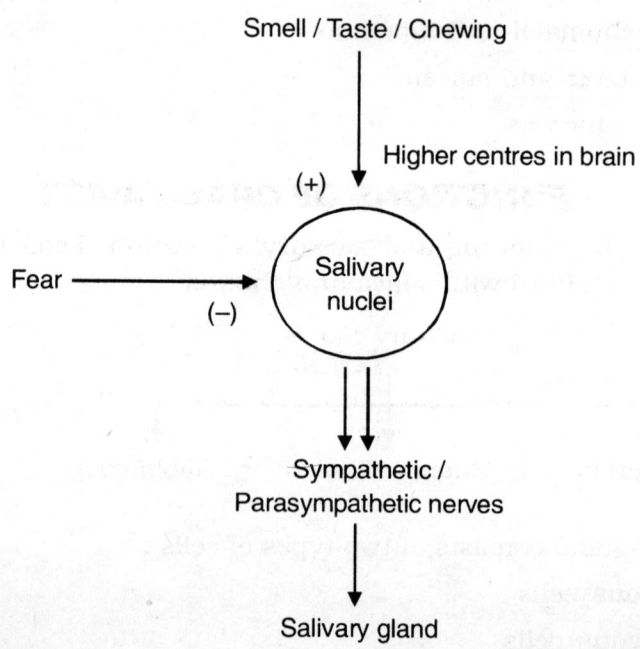

Fig. 9.4 Secretion of saliva.

Swallowing

Stage I — Oral phase – Voluntary
Stage II — Pharyngeal phase ⎫
Stage III — Oesophageal phase ⎬ → Involuntary

As swallowing occurs, a wave of peristalsis is initiated which propels the food bolus through upper oesophageal sphincter into oesophagus. The wave of contraction continues for several seconds and moves the bolus down to the lower oesophageal sphincter which relaxes to permit the entry of food into the stomach.

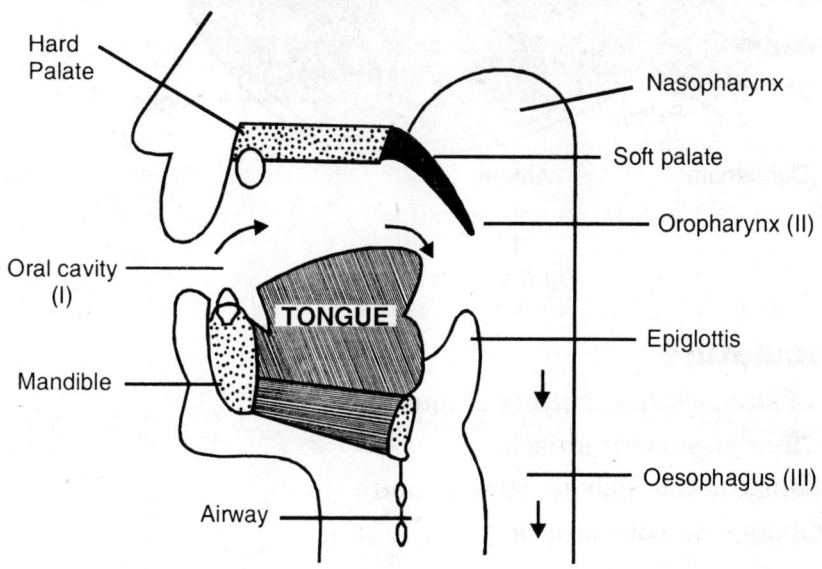

Fig. 9.5 Structures involved in swollowing.

STOMACH

It is a hollow muscular organ. It stores food temporarily for mixing, churning and kneading.

Parts of stomach

1. Fundus
2. Body
3. Pyloric

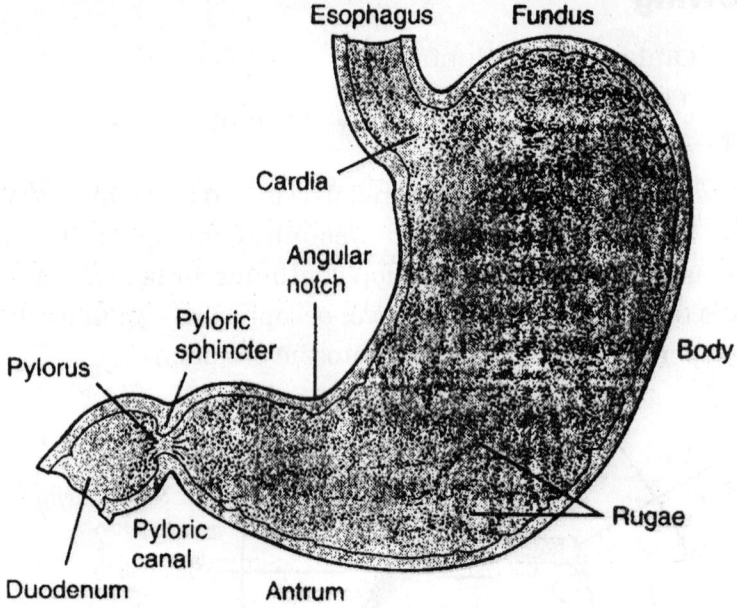

Fig. 9.6 Parts of stomach.

Musculature

Wall of stomach has 3 layers of muscle :
1. Circular smooth muscle
2. Longitudinal smooth muscle and
3. Oblique smooth muscle.

Glands

Main gastric glands –
1. Pepsinogen
2. HCl

Cardiac tubular glands — soluble mucus

Antral glands — gastrin

Pepsinogen :
1. Secreted by main gastric glands.
2. It is inactive protein which is convented into active enzyme by the action of HCl.

$$\text{Pepsinogen} \xrightarrow[\text{pH}<6]{\text{HCl}} \text{Pepsin}$$

Action of pepsin :
1. Digests protein
2. Forms soluble casein

Gastrin

1. Secreted by gastrin cells.
2. Occurs in three forms
   (a) G34
   (b) G17
   (c) G14

Action :
1. Gastric acid secretion.
2. Growth of stomach mucosa.

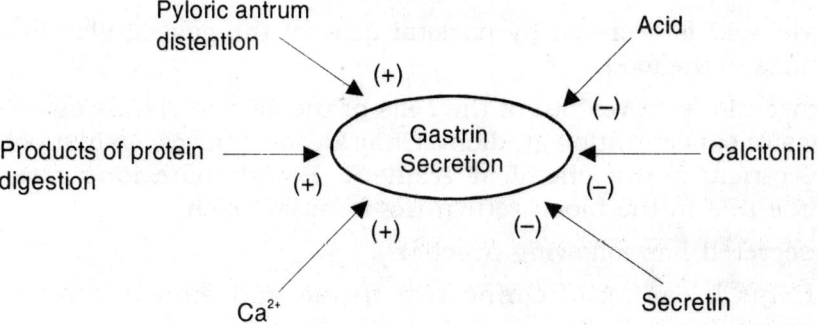

Fig. 9.7 Factors influencing gastrin secretion.

Gastric juice

The fluid secreted into the stomach by the gastric glands.
It contains :
1. Pepsinogen
2. Rennin
3. Gelatinase
4. Urease
5. Salts
6. Water
7. HCl
8. Intrinsic factor
9. Mucus

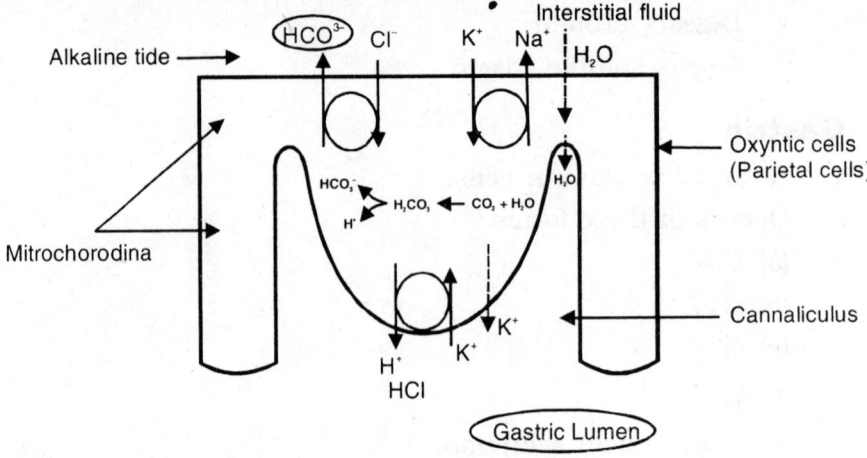

Fig. 9.8 Mechanism of secretion of gastric acid.

Gastric acid is secreted by parietal cells of the gastric glands in response to the food.

Hydrogen ions moves out of the cells of the gastric glands against a massive concentration gradient. Chloride ions moves against both an electrical and a chemical gradient. Bicarbonate ions create alkaline tide in the blood return-ing from stomach.

HCl secreted has following function :

1. Helps breaking of connective tissue and muscle fibres of ingested meat.
2. Activation of pepsinogen.

$$\text{Pepsinogen} \xrightarrow[\text{pH}<6]{\text{HCl}} \text{Pepsin}$$

3. Providing optimal condition for activity of pepsin.
4. Kills many bacteria, e.g. typhoid, cholera.

Gastric function tests :

1. Fractional test meal
2. Pentagastrin test
3. Histamine test
4. Insulin test
5. X-ray
6. Barium meal
7. Endoscopy

Regulation of gastric juice secretion : Endocrinal and nervous mechanisms combine to regulate gastric secreation.

Gastric secretion occurs in three phase :
1. Cephalic
2. Gastric
3. Intestinal

Cephalic phase : Sight, smell, taste of food, chewing
↓
Lead to vagal stimulation
↓
Secretion of gastrin

Gastric phase : Distention of stomach due to food, amino acids and peptides
↓(+)
HCl, pepsinogen, gastrin

Intestinal phase : Secretion of CCK and GIP
↓
(–)
Gastric secretion.

VOMITING

It is a protective mechanism whereby potentially toxic or noxious substances are expelled from GI tract. Metabolic alkalosis occurs on prolonged vomiting.

Vomiting is a forceful expulsion of the food from the stomach and/or intestine.

Afferents go through vagus nerve. Vomiting centre and chemoreceptor trigger zone in medulla are the site of action of these afferents. Motor impulses come via the trigeminal, facial, vagus, glossopharyngeal, hypoglossal nerves (V, VII, IX, X, XII).

SMALL INTESTINE

Digestion and absorption occurs mainly in small intestine.

Intestinal contents are mixed with the intestinal juice, parcreatic juice and bile.

Enzymes of small intestine

Enzyme	Action
Chymotrypsin	Cleaves internal peptide bonds.
Trypsin	Cleaves internal peptide bonds.
RNAase	Cleaves RNA into short fragment.
DNAase	Cleaves DNA into short fragment.
Colipase	Binds to Micelles to anchor lipase.
Amylase	Digest starch to maltose and oligo-saccharides.
Lipase	Cleaves glycerides to liberate fatty acids and glycerol.
Phospholipase A_2	Cleaves fatty acids from phospho-lipids.

Contents
1. Water
2. CCK (Cholecystokinin)
3. Neurotensin
4. Secretin
5. Somatostats
6. Lysozyme
7. Alkaline fluid
8. Mucus

A huge surface area is provided by small intestine for absorption.

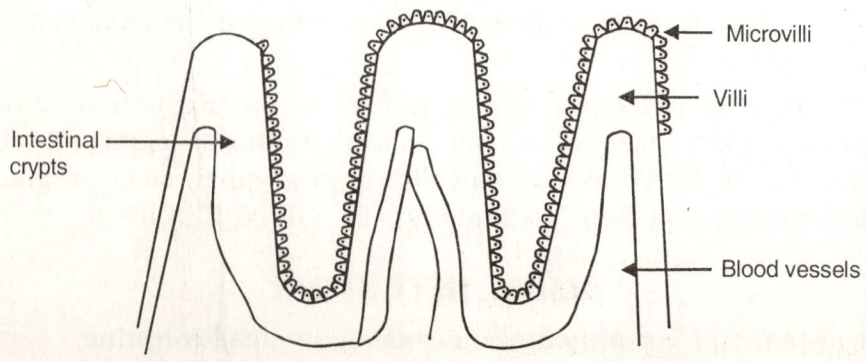

Fig. 9.9 Small intestine.

Factors responsible for large surface area are :
1. Intestinal mucosa is thrown into folds called the villi.
2. Further more the villi are also studded by small finger like projections called the microvilli.

Intestinal movements

Two types of contractions are seen in the small intestine :
1. Rhythmic
2. Peristalsis

Rhythmic contraction : Ring-like contraction occurring at regular interval.

Peristalsis : Intestinal wall distends due to food and circular constriction forms above it due to circular muscle layer contraction. Lumen below is dialated due to longitudinal muscle contraction.

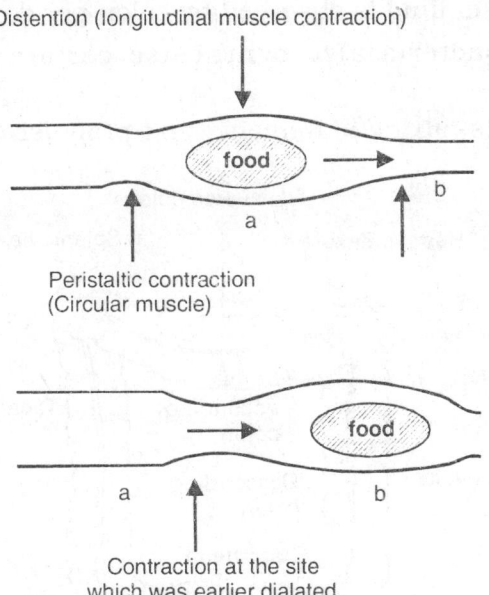

Fig. 9.10 Peristaltic movements in small intestine.

The rate at which chyme moves through the small intestine is such as that there is adequate time for absorption and digestion.

Motility of smooth muscles of small intestine is influenced by both extrinsic and intrinsic neurons and intramural plexus. Intestinal motility is enhanced by parasympathetic activity.

LARGE INTESTINE

Consists of
1. Caecum
2. Colon (Ascending, Transverse, Descending)
3. Rectum
4. Anal canal

Functions
1. To store food residues
2. Secrete mucus
3. Remaining water and electrolytes are absorbed.

Contraction
1. Peristaltic
2. Segmental

400-1000 ml of fluid is absorbed by colon per day.

Intestinal bacteria also synthesise certain vitamins such as Vit.-K.

Colon exhibits mixing movements and propulsive movements.

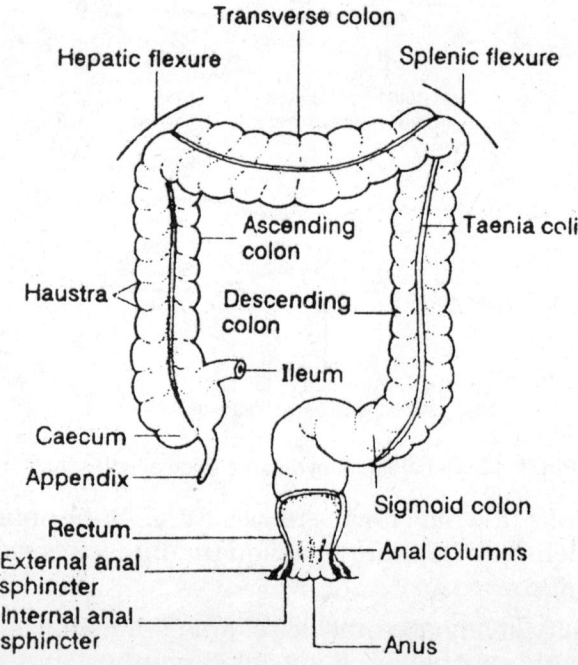

Fig. 9.11 The large intestine.

Defecation

2 types of anal sphincters are present :

1. Internal – It is involuntary.
2. External – It is voluntary.

Each day 100-150 gm of feces are eliminated.

Muscles of abdominal wall and diaphragm are also involved during defecation.

> **Defecation reflex :** Afferent impulses travel in pelvic nerves and induce reflex parasympathetic input to internal anal sphincter.

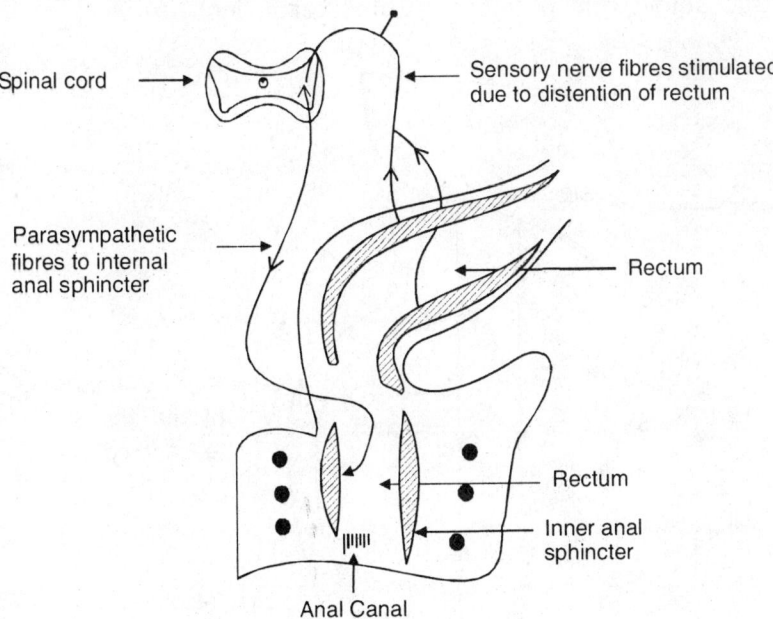

Fig. 9.12 Defecation reflex.

LIVER

It is the largest gland in the body and weighs about 1.5 kg in an adult.

Functions

1. Most of plasma proteins are synthesised.
2. Clotting factor synthesis.
3. Enzymes – SGOT, SGPT.
4. Removal of ammonia from body.
5. Synthesis of urea.

6. β oxidation.
7. Synthesis of lipoproteins saturated fatty acids.
8. Bile secretion.
9. Detoxification and protective function.

Liver secretes 500-1000 ml of bile each day. Bile is vital for the processing of fats by small intestine. It is stored and concentrated in the gall bladder which contracts to deliver bile to duodenum after meal.

Bile constituents are as follows :

1. Na, Ca^{2+}
2. HCO_3^-, Cl^-
3. Bile acids, bile pigments, cholesterol, lecithin.

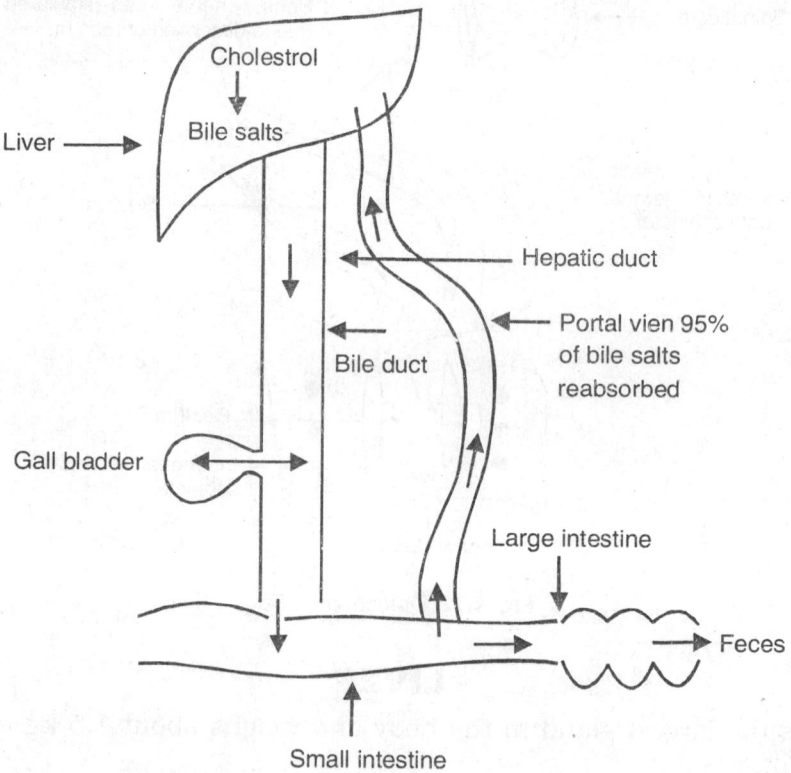

Fig. 9.13 Enterohepatic circulation of bile salts.

Enterohepatic circulation

90-95% of total bile salts, which enter the duodenum are reabsorbed actively from the terminal ileum into the portal vein and come back to the liver.

Liver bile is light golden yellow with 97% of water and 2-4% solids as compared to gall bladder bile which is almost black in colour with 89% water and 10-12% solids.

The substances which increase the rate of bile secretion are called choleretic, e.g., bile acids.

Functions of bile

1. Acid neutralization.
2. Helps in digestion and absorption of fats and absorption of fat soluble vitamins with the help of bile salt.
3. Many drugs, bile pigments are excreted.

Bile secretion is under the nervous and humoral regulation.

Cholagogues are substances that cause contraction of gall bladder, e.g. fatty acids.

Gall Bladder

It stores bile, reduces its alkalinity and controls the flow of bile following a meal.

Liver function test

1. To check any damage to liver.
2. Diagnosing hepatic insufficiency.

Test include :

1. Albumin / globulin ratio.
2. Test for coagulability of blood.
3. Estimation of plasma proteins by electrophoreses.
4. Liver enzyme estimation. SGOT / SGPT.
5. Blood urea / ammonia.

DIET

Diet is the selection of foods eaten by an individual.

A *balanced diet* is essential for maintainence of good health. A balanced diet is one which contains all nutrients in adequate amounts to maintain a good health.

Nutrient

Any substance that is utilized or absorbed to promote the activities of cells and, in turn, the function of whole body.

They include :
1. Carbohydrate
2. Proteins
3. Fats
4. Vitamins
5. Minerals
6. Water

Essential nutrients : Those nutrients that cannot be made by the body and therefore required in the diet.

Hunger and appetite are important regulator of food intake. Feeding and satiety centres are located in the hypothalamus.

DIGESTION AND ABSORPTION IN THE GIT

Digestion
Breaking of complex substances into simpler ones.

Absorption
Process of transport of products of digestion into the epithelial cells that line the GI tract and from their to blood or lymph draining the tract.

Carbohydrates
Daily intake of carbohydrate contains :
1. Monosacchrides, e.g., glucose, fructose, galactose.
2. Dissacchrides, e.g., sucrose, lactose, maltose.
3. Polysacchrides, e.g., starch, cellulose, glycogens.

Digestion :
1. Salivary amylase converts starch to maltose.
2. In stomach HCl hydrolyses sucrose.
3. In duodenum α amylase converts all forms of starch into maltose.
4. In small intestine :
   (a) Maltose → 2 glucose
   (b) Lactose → glucose + galactose

Absorption : Glucose, galactose and fructose are absorbed largely in the duodenum and upper jejunum.

Glucose and galactose are taken up into the epithelial cells against their concentration gradient by sodium-dependent cotransport mechanism. Sodium gradient that drives this transport is maintained by $Na^+ - K^+$ ATP-ase. At the basolateral membrane the monosaccharide leaves the intestinal epithelial cells by facilitated diffusion. Sodium independent facilitated diffusion helps in fructose absorption.

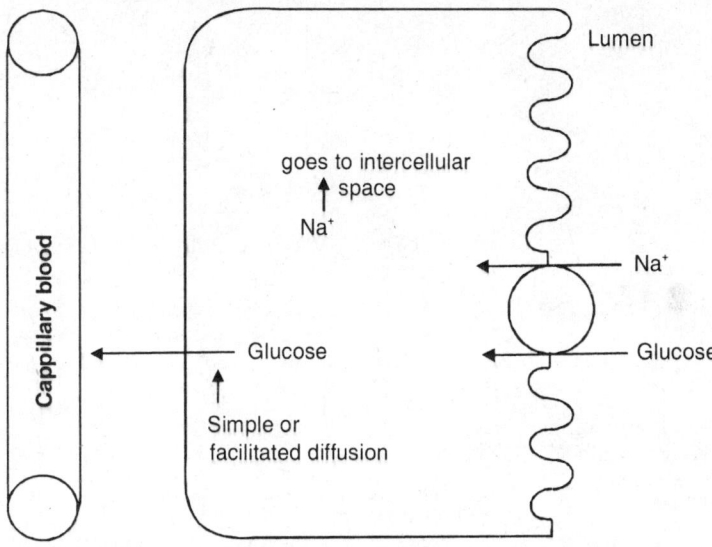

Fig. 9.14 Glucose absorption from intestinal site.

Fats (Lipids)

Classification : Simple fats, e.g., palmitic acid, stearic acid. Compound fats, e.g., phospholipids, lecithin. Associated fats, e.g., steroids.

Digestion and absorption :

1. Salivary lipase digests much of triglycerides.
2. Stomach contains lipase which helps in lipolysis.
3. In small intestine, pancreatic lipase and bile salts help in fat digestion.
4. The product of fat digestion are incorporated into micelles along with bile salts, lecithins, cholestrol and fat-soluble vitamins. In this way they are brought close to enterocyte membrane and the fatty components of the micelle diffuse into the cells. Bile salts are recycled and fats are reprocessed by the smooth endoplasmic reticulum to form chylomicrons. These are exocytosed across the baso-lateral cell membrane and enter the lacteals of the villi.

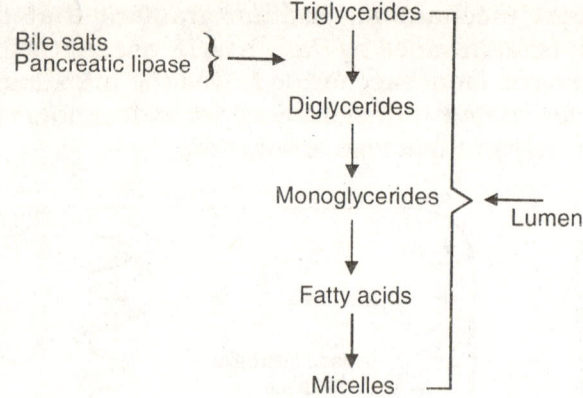

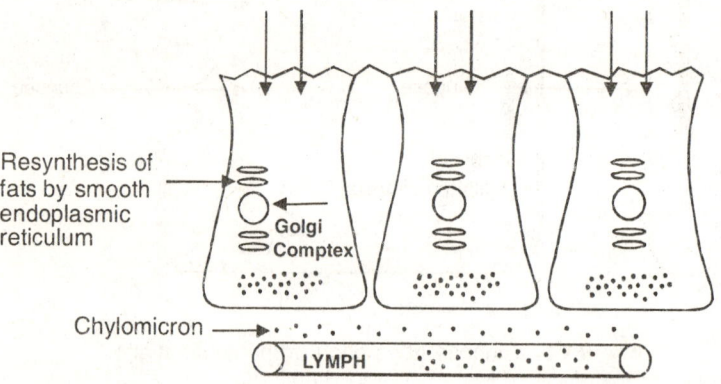

Fig. 9.15 Summary of digestion and absorption of lipids.

Proteins

Digestion : In stomach, pepsin hydrolyze the bonds between amino acids.

Duodenum contains trypsin and small intestine contains peptidase.

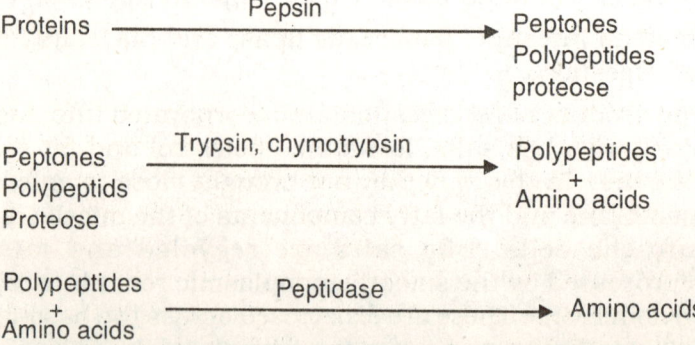

Absorption : Amino acids are absorbed at the brush border of the intestinal epithelial cells by sodium dependent co-transport. There are three different type of transporter for neutral, acidic and basic amino acid. A fourth transporter exists for proline and hydroxyproline. After entering the enterocytes amino acids pass across the basolateral surface into the blood capillaries of the villus and from their to portal vein.

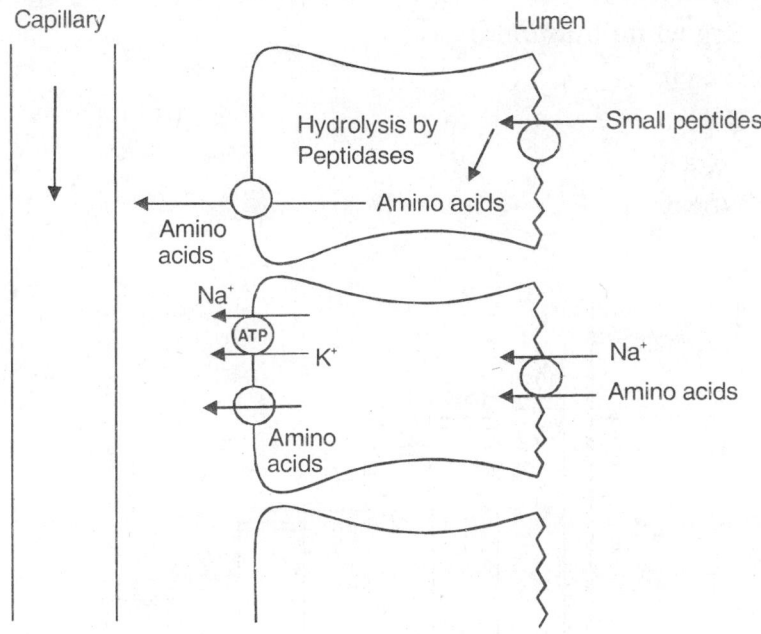

Fig. 9.16 Absorption of amino acids.

ABSORPTION OF FLUIDS / ELECTROLYTES / VITAMINS

Most of fluid is absorbed from the small and large intestine. Quite less amount around 50-100 ml leaves the body with feces. Digestive juices account for 7-10 litres of fluid to gastrointestinal tract. Approximately 2-3 litres of fluids are ingested. This total fluid comes out to 9-13 litres.

Small intestine absorbs around 8500 ml / day. The active transport of sodium and nutrient are followed by amino movement and osmosis (absorption of water). Life threatening diarrhoea can occur if the above mechanism of absorption does not occurs.

Water soluble vitamins are absorbed by facilitated transport. Fat soluble vitamins are absorbed along with the products of fat digestion; vitamin B_{12} absorption needs a specific uptake process involving intrinsic factor.

BIOLOGICAL VALUE (B.V.)

Biological value measures amount of protein nitrogen that is retained by body from a given amount of nitrogen that has been consumed. Whey proteins have BV value of 104 which is considerably higher than the BV for milk protein, soy protein, and egg white protein.

1. Whey protein
2. Whole egg
3. Egg white (Albumin)
4. Casein
5. Rice
6. Soya
7. Wheat

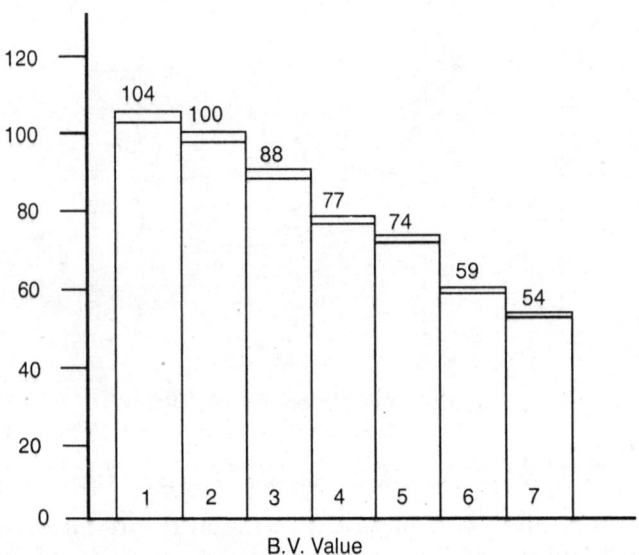

Fig. 9.17 Biological value of some common food proteins.

10
THE INTEGUMENTORY SYSTEM

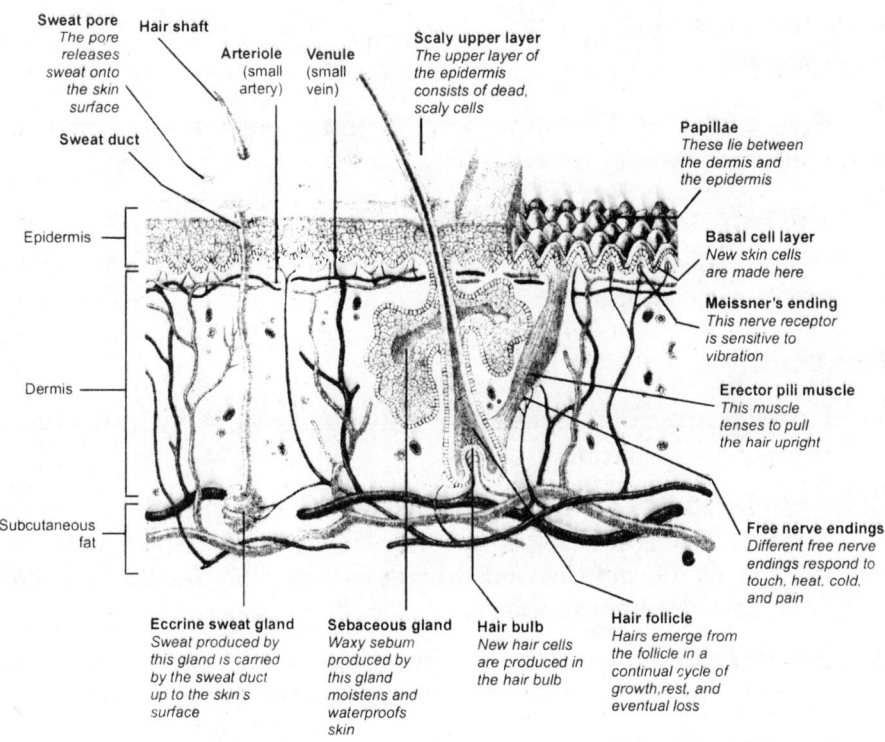

Fig. 10.1 Skin and hair.

INTRODUCTION

A group of tissues performing a specific function is known as an organ. Under integumentary system following organs are involved. Skin and its derivatives like glands, hairs, nails and nerve endings.

THE SKIN

It is an organ since it has different tissues that are joined to perform specific activities.

In adult skin covers about 2 m² area and weighs about 4-5 kg.

Dermatology

It is the science dealing with the diagnosis and treatment of skin disorders.

Anatomical aspects

Skin consists of two parts :
1. Epidermis
2. Dermis

Epidermis : The superficial, thinner portion composed of epithelial tissue.

Dermis : The deeper, thicker, connective tissue.

Deeper to dermis is superficial fascia which is made up of areolar and adipose tissues.

Functions

1. **Protection** from physical abrasion, bacteria, dehydration and ultraviolet radiation.
2. **Regulation of body temperature :** The evaporation of sweat from skin surface helps to lower down body temperature to normal which gets raised during exercise or due to external environmental temperature.
3. **Sensation :** A number of nerve endings and receptors are in the skin that detect stimuli relating to temperature, touch, etc.
4. **Vitamin D synthesis :** Synthesis of vitamin D begins with activation of a precursor molecule in the skin by UV rays in sunlight.
5. **Immunity**
6. **Reservoir of blood :** The skin dermis carry 8-10% of total blood flow in resting adult. Increase in blood flow occurs in exercise, etc.

GLANDS

Several kinds of glands are associated with the skin :

1. Sebaceous glands
2. Sweat glands
3. Mammary glands
4. Ceruminous glands

Sebaceous glands

These glands secrete an oily substance called sebum, which is a mixture of fats, cholesterol, proteins and inorganic salts. The secreting portions of the glands lie in the dermis and open into the necks of hair follicles or directly onto a skin surface.

Sebum helps keep hair from drying and becoming brittle, prevents excessive evaporation of water from the skin, keeps the skin soft and pliable, and inhibits the growth of certain bacteria.

Sweat glands

These are of two types :

Eccrine sweat glands : These are distributed throughout the skin except margins of lips, nail beds of the fingers and toes, glans penis, glans clitoris, labia minora and eardrums are most numerous in the soles and palms. Their secretory portion lies in the subcutaneous layer.

Apocrine sweat glands : Found mainly in skin of the axilla, pubic region and areolae of breasts. Their secretory portion lies in the subcutaneous or dermis layer and the excretory ducts open into hair follicles. These begin to function at puberty and they produce a more viscous secretion than eccrine sweat glands.

Sweat is a mixture of water, ions (Na^+ and Cl^-), urea, uric acid, amino acids, ammonia, glucose, lactic acid and ascorbic acid.

Mammary glands

These are specialised sweat glands that produce milk. A mammary gland consists of 15-20 lobes separated by adipose tissue. In each lobe are several smaller compartments called lobules, composed of grape-like clusters of milk-secreting glands termed alveoli, which are surrounded by myoepithelial cells whose contraction helps propel milk towards the nipples.

Ceruminous glands

These are the modified sweat glands present in ears, and produce a waxy secretion. Their excretory ducts open directly on to the surface of the external auditory canal or into ducts of sebaceous glands. The combined secretion of the ceruminous and sebaceous glands is called cerumen.

BODY TEMPERATURE REGULATION

The environment temperature may be –20 °C or 50 °C but mouth temperature is about 37 °C in all cases. This shows that there exists a mechanism of thermal regulation.

The purpose of temperature regulation is to provide the tissues a *microenvironment* at the optimal temperature. The temperature of blood is regulated.

Core temperature – It is the temperature of organs deep inside the body which is quite matching with that of blood.

Shell temperature – It is the temperature of the superficial part of the body.

The core body temperature shows a diurnal variation. The temperature is higher during the day as compared to night. In women, the body temperature shows cyclic variation synchronous with the menstrual cycle.

The regulation of body temperature depends on a balance of heat gain and heat loss.

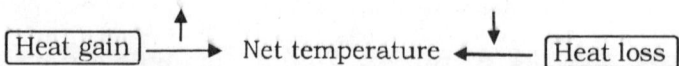

The gain in the body heat due to increased heat production is a direct method of heat gain. These methods can be due to shivering, exercise, metabolic rate increase, etc.

Decrease in heat loss due to cutaneous vasoconstriction, reduced air movement, reduced surface area also contribute to the heat gain.

When there is increased heat production certain processes takes place which lead to increased heat loss to maintain a neutral body temperature. Such processes are cutaneous vasodilatation, sweating, cooler environment, or increased surface area.

Decrease in heat conservation also helps in heat loss to maintain body temperature. Such processes can be clothing, woolen are used in cold surroundings to conserve heat.

Temperature regulatory mechanism

1. Thermosensitive areas.
2. Central nervous system involvement.
3. The effect.

Thermosensitive areas : There are many thermosensitive areas in the body which are involved in thermoregulation. There are also some nerve endings specially acting as thermoreceptors; certain thermosensitive neurons have also been described.

Central nervous system involvement : Specially hypothalamus is the central processor for the thermoregulation. Anterior hypothalamus initiates heat dissipation whereas posterior hypothalamus acts as a heat conservation and production machinery.

The effect : The implementation of thermoregulation is via heat dissipation or heat production and conservation mechanisms.

**THE BEST
TRANQUILIZER IS A CLEAR CONSCIENCE.**

11
THE RESPIRATORY SYSTEM

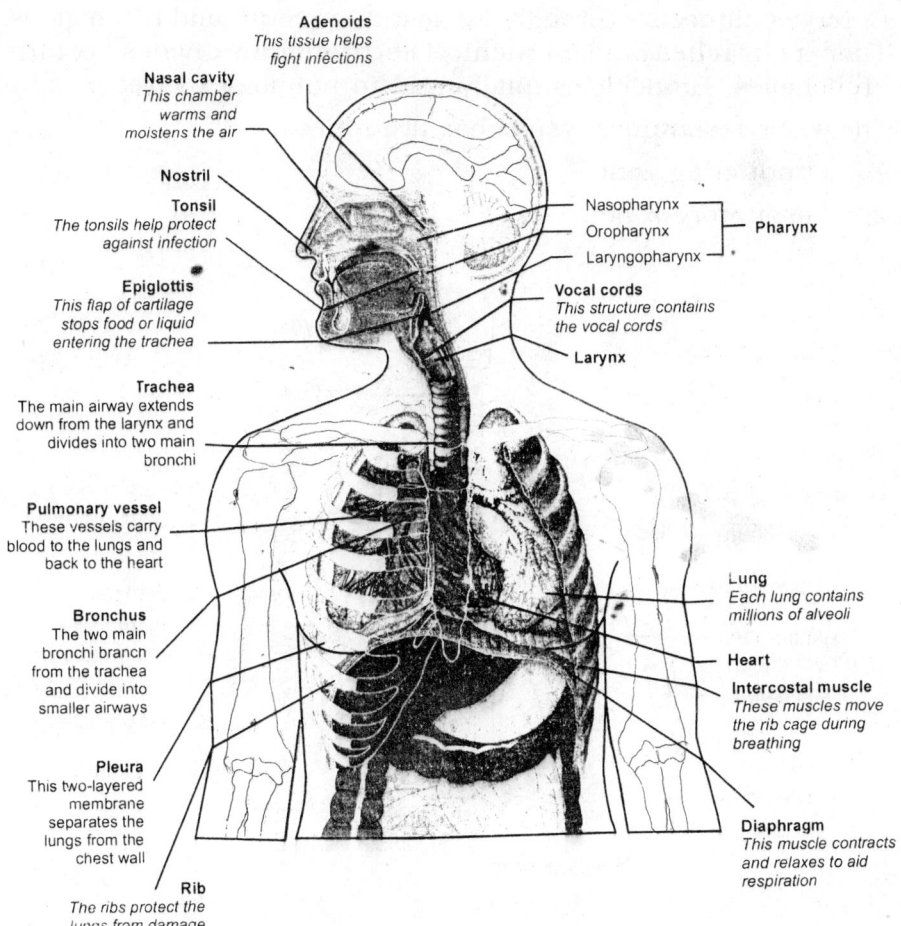

Fig. 11.1 Respiratory system.

INTRODUCTION

Respiratory system functions primarily to provide oxygen to the tissues and to remove the carbon dioxide. Thus, it has following functions :

1. Pulmonary ventilation and its regulation.
2. Diffusion of oxygen and carbon dioxide between the alveoli and the blood and supply of oxygen to the tissues and removal of carbon dioxide from different parts of the body.
3. Helps regulate blood pH.

ANATOMY

Respiratory passage

Entery of air occurs through the nose and mouth and reach glotis. Then to trachea and bronchi. The bronchus divides to form bronchioles. Bronchioles finally lead to pulmonary alveoli.

The whole respiratory system has two zones :
1. Conducting zone
2. Respiratory zone

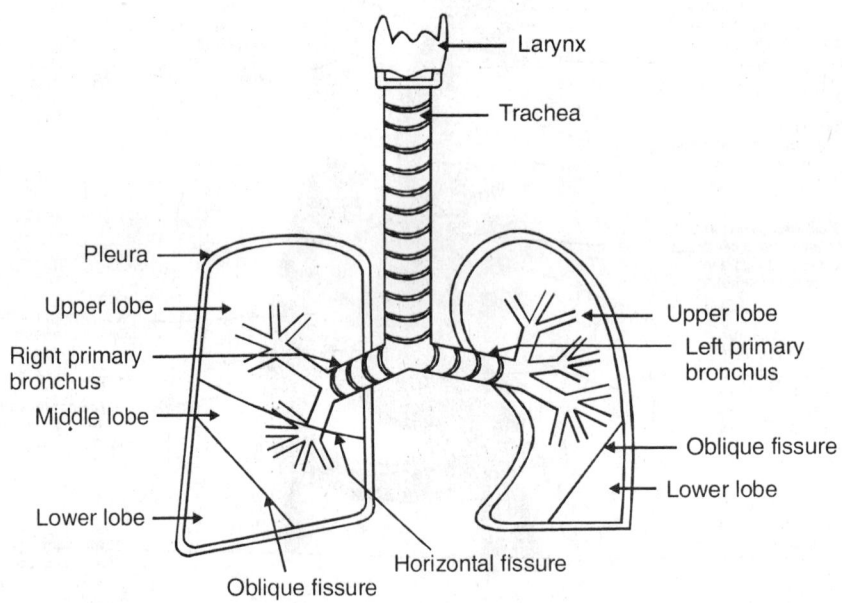

Fig. 11.2 Trachea and lungs.

Branching of the bronchial tree

Treachea
↓
Primary bronchi

↓
Secondary bronchi
↓
Tertiary bronchi
↓
Bronchioles
↓
Terminal bronchioles
↓
Respiratory bronchioles
↓
Alveolar sacs

In normal condition air flows through the respiratory passage very easily.

NERVOUS CONTROL

Sympathetic nerves

Cause dilatation of bronchioles. But the direct control is weak.

Parasympathetic nerves

Cause bronchoconstriction. Besides this, parasympathetic nerves also cause increased bronchial secretion.

LOCAL FACTORS

Several local factors i.e. substances formed in the lungs cause bronchoconstriction. Example are histamine and slow reactive substances of anaphylaxis.

One of the most important thing for respiratory passage is its patency i.e. keeping it open. Trachea is prevented from collapsing due to multiple ring cartilages. In bronchial wall less extensive cartilage also maintain rigidity. The bronchioles are kept expended by trans-pulmonary pressures.

In all areas of bronchi and trachea where no cartilage is present is occupied by smooth muscle.

Respiratory bronchioles i.e. the most terminal bronchioles contain only a few smooth muscles.

RESPIRATORY MEMBRANE

It seprates air in the alveoli from the blood in capillaris of lung. It is formed of alveolar wall and capillary wall and interstitial space.

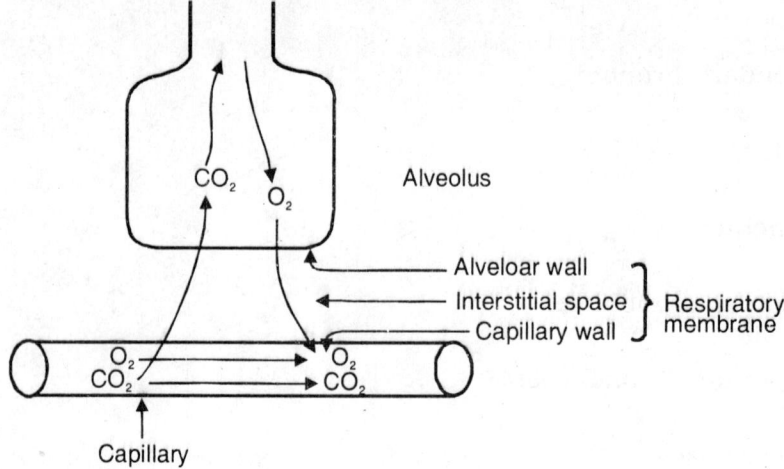

Fig. 11.3 Respiratory membrane.

Diffusing capacity of respiratory membrane

The amount of gas which diffuses through the membrane each minute for a pressure difference of 1 mmHg.

NOSE

Nose is the point of entry of air. It humidifies and filters the air besides warming it.

The most important function of nose is in filtering out of large particles by turbulent precipitation.

PLEURA

The *lungs* are invested by two layers of pleura :
  1. **Parietal layer**
  2. **Visceral layer**

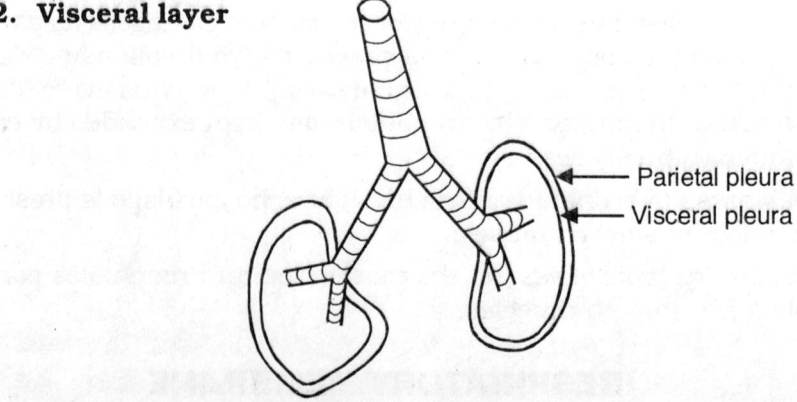

Fig. 11.4 Lung showing the pleura.

THE RESPIRATORY UNIT

Respiratory bronchiole
   +
Alveolar ducts
   +
Atria
   +
Alveoli

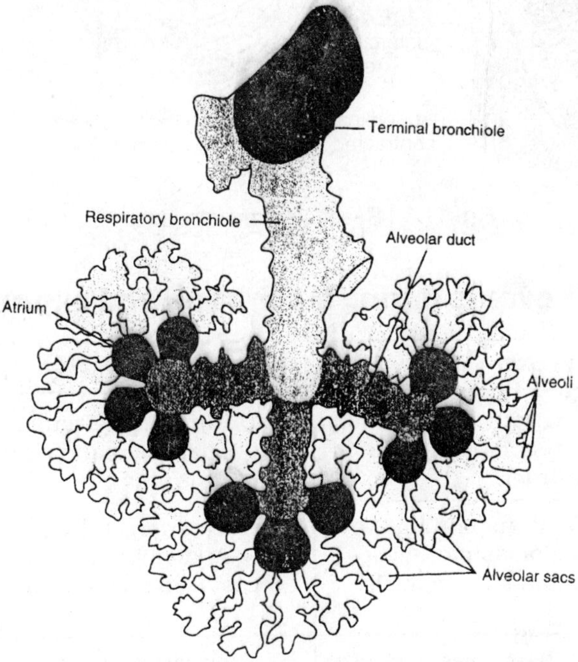

Fig. 11.5 The respiratory unit.

RESPIRATORY MOVEMENTS

The normal breathing at rest consists of inspiration and expiration.

Inspiration

Inhalation of air during which thorax is enlarged by rib movements and diaphragmatic movements. A-P and vertical diameters increase. External intercostals contracts.

Expiration

Exhalation of air during which anterior abdominal wall muscles contract. Expiration is a passive process as compared to inspiration which is an active process.

Following diagram depicts contraction and expansion of thoracic cage during expiration and inspiration respectively.

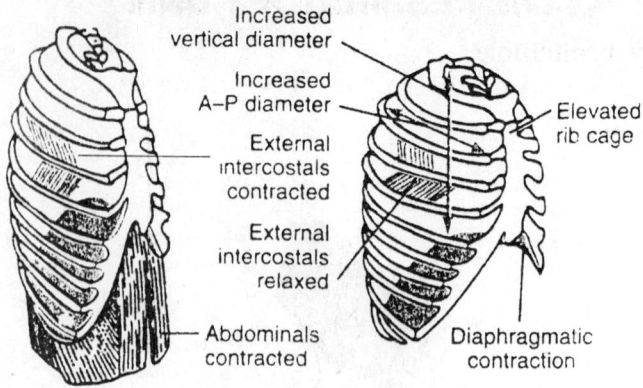

Fig. 11.6 Respiratory movements.

Summary of events during inspiration and expiration

Inspiration	Expiration
1. During normal quiet inspiration — Diaphragm and external intercostals countract.	1. During normal quiet expiration — Diaphram and external intercostals relax.
2. During forceful inspiration — Sternocleidomastoid, scalenes, and pectoralis minor also contract.	2. During forceful expiration — Abdominal and internal intercostal muscles also contract.
3. Thoracic cavity increases in size and volume of lung increases.	3. Thoracic cavity decreases in size and lungs are reduced in volume.

ALVEOLAR PRESSURE

Alveolar pressure is the pressure of air inside the lung alveoli.

Transpulmonary pressure

It is the pressure difference between the alveolar pressure and pleural pressure.

Pleural pressure

It is the pressure of the fluid in the narrow space between the pleura of the visceral and parietal layers of pleura.

Alveolar pressure
↑
Transpulmonary pressure
↓
Pleural pressure

PULMONARY VOLUMES

Tidal volume
The volume of air inspired and expired with each normal breath (normal 500 ml).

Inspiratory reserve volume
The maximum extra volume of air which can be inspired over and above normal tidal volume (normal - 3 litres).

Expiratory reserve volume
The maximal volume of air which can be expired after a normal tidal expiration (normal - 1.1 litres).

Residual volume
It is the volume of air which remains in the lungs after the most forceful expiration (normal - 1.2 litres).

Closing volume
The lung volume above the residual volume at which the airways in the lower, dependent part of lungs begin to close off.

PULMONARY CAPACITIES

The inspiratory capacity
Maximal volume of air which can be inspired after completing tidal expiration.

The vital capacity
It is the maximal volume of air which can be expelled from the lungs forcefully following maximal inspiration.

VC = Inspiratory Reserve Volume + Tidal Volume + Expiratory Reserve Volume

Normal – 4.8 litres in males. 3.2 litres in females.

Functional residual capacity
The amount of air that remains in the lungs at the end of normal expiration.

FRC = Reserve Volume + Expiratary Reserve Volume.

Normal – 2.5 litres.

Total lung capacity

It is the maximum volume to which the lungs can be expanded with the greatest possible effort.

TLC = Vital capacity + Residual Volume.

Normal – 6 litres.

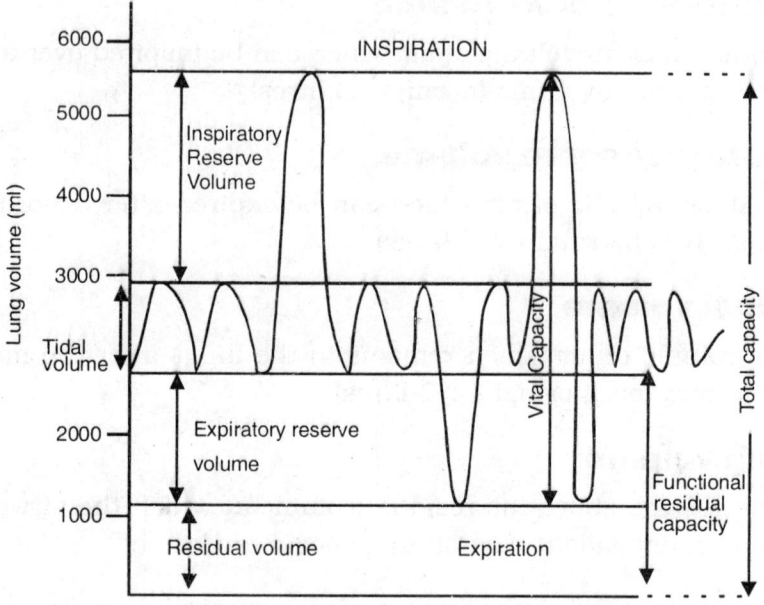

Fig. 11.7 Pulmonary volumes and capacities.

DYNAMIC PULMONARY VOLUME

Forced vital capacity

Vital capacity recorded on a spirograph at a known speed, volume of air expelled is timed.

FVC components

1. FEV_1 (Forced Expiratory Volume in one sec.)
2. FEV_2 (Forced Expiratory Volume in two sec.)
3. FEV_3 (Forced Expiratory Volume in three sec.)

SPIROMETRY

It is the simple method for studying pulmonary ventilation. It records the volume movement of air into and out of the lungs. A spirometer helps in recording pulmonary ventilation. A spirometer consist of a floating drum, oxygen chamber, counter balancing weights, recording drum and mouthpiece.

COMPLIANCE OF THE LUNGS

Compliance is the extent to which the lungs expand for each unit of increase in transpulmonary pressure. It is expressed as litres / cm H_2O.

It is measured by measuring intrapleural pressures at different lung volumes. Each curve is recorded by changing transpulmonary pressure is small steps. We get two curves :

1. Inspiratory curve
2. Expiratory curve

Compliance is determined by elastic forces of the lung tissue and that caused by surface tension of the fluid lining the inside walls of alveoli.

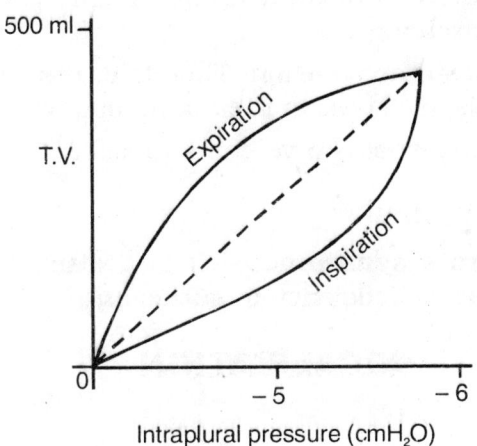

Fig. 11.8 Compliance diagram of lung.

SURFACTANT

It is a mixture of protein lipid complexes. It greatly reduces the surface tension of the water. Type-II alveolar epithelial cells secrete this surfactant.

Components of surfactant

1. Dipalmitoylphosphatidylcholine.
2. Calcium ions.
3. Certain proteins.
4. Neutral lipids.

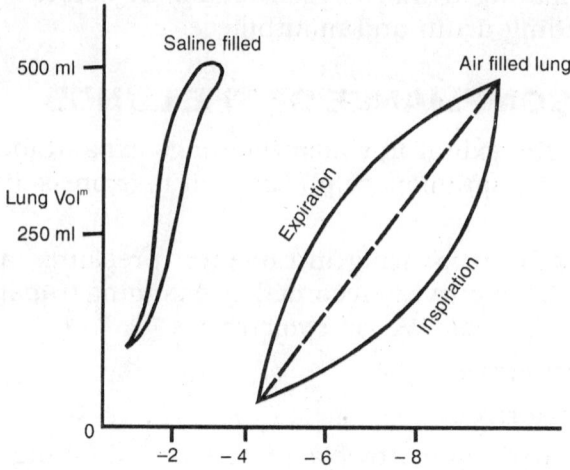

Fig. 11.9 Surfactant.

Surface tension due to surfactant keeps the alveoli dry and thus helps in gaseous exchange.

Saline reduces the surface tension. Therefore, the curve obtained after using saline is as shown in the above diagram.

On adding saline the whole curve shifts to 'left'.

Clinical importance

Respiratory distress syndrome — It is a disease seen in the newborn infant due to deficiency of surfactant.

VOCALIZATION

Speech involves :
1. Respiratory system
2. Nervous control centres
3. Respiratory control centres
4. Articulation
5. Phonation
6. Resonance

Phonation

Phonation for vocalization is produced by the large vibrating elements called vocal cords.

Articulation

It is achieved by mouth structures. It includes lips, tongue and soft palate.

Resonance

Resonance is an important part of voice production. It is produced by mouth, nose, chest cavity.

COUGH REFLEX

A very slight touch to bronchi and trachea due to foreign matter or other irritation can initiate cough reflex. This occurs because the bronchi and trachea are quit sensitive. Vagus nerve takes afferent impulses from the respiratory tract which leads to this autonomic reflex.

RESPIRATORY QUOTIENT

It is the ratio of CO_2 production to O_2 utilization.

Respiratory quotient is used to estimate fat and carbohydrate utilization. When fat is oxidized in the body on an average 68 molecules of carbon dioxide molecules are formed for each 100 molecules of oxygen consumed. Therefore, respiratory quotient of fat is 0.68. Carbohydrates have respiratory quotient of 1.0. Proteins have 0.80.

COMPOSITION OF INSPIRED AND EXPIRED AIR

Gas diffusion

Diffusion is the process by which simple molecules freely move among each other. All the gases that participate in respiratory processes move by diffusion.

Atmospheric air has following gases in following partial pressure and percentage :

Gases	Partial Pressure
O_2	159 mmHg
CO_2	0.3 mmHg
N_2	595 mmHg
H_2O	3.7 mmHg

Percentage of different gases in air is as follow :

Gases	Percentage
O_2	20.84%
CO_2	0.04%
N_2	78%
H_2O	0.50

When the air reaches the alveolus the proportion is different:

Gases	Partial Pressure	Percentage
O_2	120 mm Hg	16%
CO_2	27 mm Hg	4%
N_2	566 mm Hg	75%
H_2O	47 mm Hg	7%

*Arterial PO_2 decreses in inspired air at high altitude.

Factors determining the pressure of dissolved gas in the fluid

Two factors determine the pressure — first is its concentration and second is solubility coefficient of the gas.

$$\text{Pressure} = \frac{\text{Concentration of dissolved gas}}{\text{Solubility coefficient}}$$

Diffusion of gas between the gas phase in the alveoli and the dissolved phase in the pulmonary blood depends upon the net diffusion.

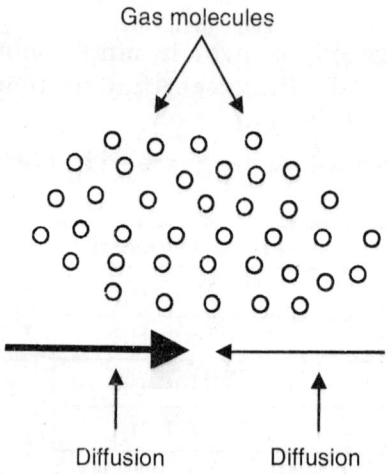

Fig. 11.10 Gas diffusion.

Net diffusion is in the direction of big arrow, since the diffusion in right direction is more.

RESPIRATION CONTROL

Respiratory control is under neural and chemical mechanisms.

Neurogenic regulation

The respiratory centre has several neurons located in pons and medulla oblongata. The respiratory center is divided into three collection of nerves :

1. Dorsal respiratory group
2. Ventral respiratory group
3. Pneumotaxic center

Dorsal respiratory group : It control the inspiration and respiratory rhythm.

Ventral respiratory group : It controls both inspiration and expiration.

Pneumotaxic center : It limits the duration of inspiration and increases the respiratory rate.

Chemical regulation

Carbon dioxide or excess of hydrogen ions in blood act directly on the respiratory center. Whereas oxygen acts through chemoreceptors located in the carotid and aortic bodies.

TRANSPORT OF OXYGEN AND CARBON DIOXIDE

The transport of gases between the lungs and body tissues is one of the function of blood.

Oxygen transport

Deoxygenated blood returning to the lungs contain CO_2 dissolved in plasma. Oxygen does not dissolve easily in water and, therefore, little is in dissolved state. 98% of O_2 is transported in chemical combination with haemoglobin inside red blood cells. Oxygen and haemoglobin combine to form oxyhaemoglobin.

$$Hb + O_2 \rightleftharpoons HbO_2$$

Reduced + Oxygen haemoglobin   Oxyhaemoglobin

Where the partial pressure of oxygen is relatively high, as occuring in the lung, haemoglobin picks up oxygen to form oxyhaemoglobin and blood leaves the lung with its haemoglobin virtually saturated with oxygen.

Affinity is such that even blood perfusing those areas of the lungs with a low ventilation/perfusion ratio, where partial pressure of oxygen is less than 100 mmHg is almost saturated with oxygen.

Deoxygenation of blood in the tissues cause the blood to become considerably darker in color than arterial blood. Thus, the haemoglobin of mixed venous blood is still some 70% saturated with oxygen and the blood contains about 14 ml of oxygen per 100 ml.

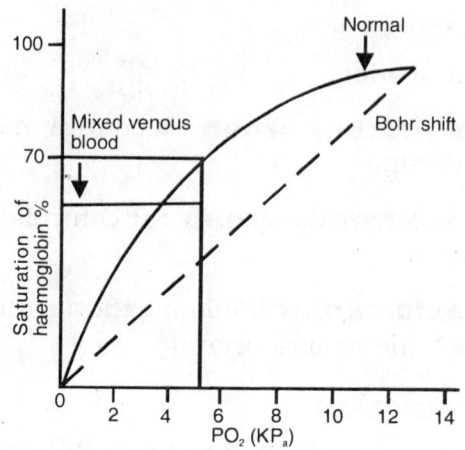

Fig. 11.11 Oxygen transport.

Haemoglobin has a property of its relationship with oxygen. Thus, under conditions found locally in highly active tissues the position of dislocation curve shifts to the right, referred as Bohr effect (Bhor shift).

The enhanced release of oxygen helps to maintain the increased metabolic demands.

Fetal haemoglobin has it dissociation curve to left of that of adult haemoglobin.

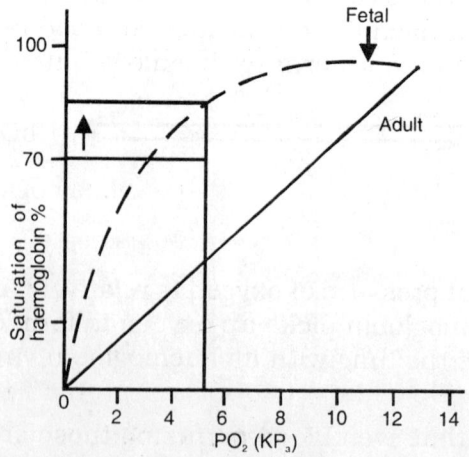

Fig. 11.12 The haemoglobin dissociation curve.

Carbon dioxide transport

As compared to oxygen which is not a soluble gas, CO_2 is highly soluble.

Haemoglobin has a role in carbon dioxide transport; about 23% of carbon dioxide produced by respiring cells is carried by pigment in the form of carbaminohaemoglobin. About 70% of carbon dioxide is carried by blood. Only 7% is carried simply as dissolved gas.

Partial pressure gradients also determine the direction of gas movement across the cell membrane.

Bicarbonate ions are formed from carbon dioxide; this is promoted within red blood cells by the enzyme carbonic anhydrase.

Carbonic acid is initially formed and weakly dissociates into bicarbonate and hydrogen ions; thus raising their concentration within the red blood cells. Since this raise in the availability promotes the reformation of carbonic acid and promotes its dissociation back into carbon dioxide

$$H^+ + Hb \rightarrow HHb$$
$$CO_2 + H_2O$$
$$\downarrow\downarrow$$
$$H_2CO_3$$
(Carbonic acid)
$$\downarrow\downarrow$$
in RBCs / plasma
$$HCO_3^- + H^+$$

The electrical imbalance of plasma produced by the diffusion of bicarbonate ions out of red blood cells is corrected by the influx of other negatively charged ions, in fact chloride ions into the blood cells. This is known as *chloride shift*.

The buffering of hydrogen ions and the efflux of most of the bicarbonate ions prevent acid base disturbance. When the blood reaches the lung the process is reversed.

Carbon dioxide dissolved in plasma and within blood cells will diffuse across the alveo-capillary membranes reducing its partial pressure in blood.

As there is in the partial pressure of blood, CO_2 will be released from carbaminohaemoglobin.

As CO_2 is removed from the blood, the dissociation of carbonic acid to carbon dioxide and water will be promoted.

This in turn will favour the formation of more carbonic acid from the bicarbonates and hydrogen ions.

$$HCO_3^- + H^+$$
$$\uparrow\downarrow$$

$$H_2CO_3$$
(Carbonic acid)
$$\updownarrow$$
$$CO_2 + H_2O$$
(Diffuses into the alveoli)

This whole process is facilitated by the enzyme carbonic anhydrase and it ensures that carbon dioxide is excreted.

On diffusion of the bicarbonate ions, chloride ions move into the plasma. So that clinical balance is maintained.

Thus, carbon dioxide carriage by blood is very different from oxygen transport.

At physiological values there is no sigmoid-shaped relationship between the partial pressure of carbon dioxide and the volume of gas being carried which would be analogous to that of the oxygen-haemoglobin dissociation curve.

Haldane effect : An increase in CO_2 in the blood causes O_2 to split from haemoglobin. In the presence of O_2, less carbon dioxide binds to haemoglobin. This reaction is the reverse of Bohr effect and it is known as *halden effect*.

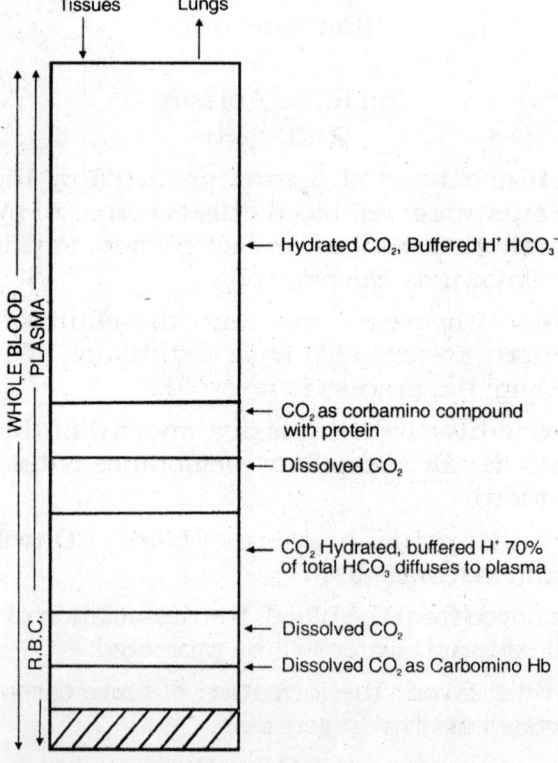

Fig. 11.13 Summary of CO_2 transport in the blood.

GAS EXCHANGE BETWEEN BLOOD AND TISSUES

The blood and lung, the blood and the tissues require presence of favourable pressure gradient for proper exchange of gases to take place.

The partial pressure of oxygen within the cells is relatively low around 40 mmHg, because the cells utilize the oxygen. This is lower than that of arterial blood perfusing the tissues (100 mmHg), so a gradient exists for oxygen transfer.

As in the lungs, equilibration between the two compartments occurs and venous blood leaves the tissues with oxygen partial pressure around 5.3 Kpa.

Carbon dioxide production takes place continuously in the cells and its partial pressure in intracellular fluid is higher at 45 mmHg as compared to arterial blood at 40 mmHg. Again, equilibration will occur so venous blood will have an average partial pressure of CO_2 around 6 Kpa. Smaller pressure gradient is required to transfer adequate amount of this CO_2. Rise in CO_2 content will generate more carbonic acid and this may create a problem but this is avoided by homeostatic regulation of the partial pressure of CO_2 in arterial blood.

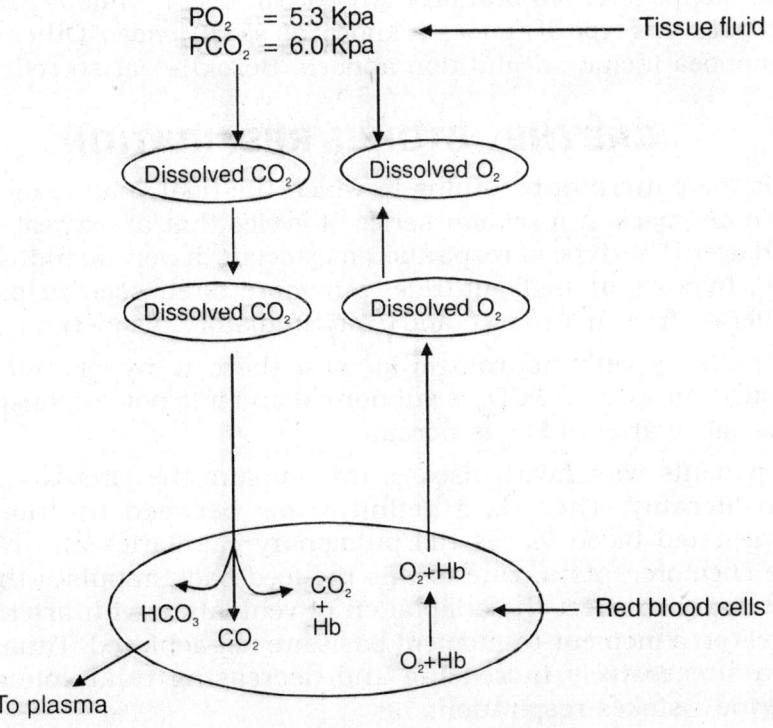

Gas exchange between blood and tissues occurs according to partial pressure of gases.

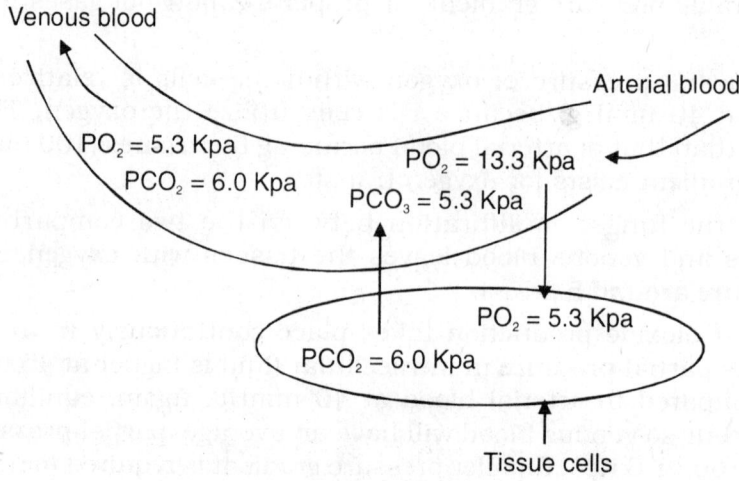

Fig. 11.14 Equilibration of blood and tissue gases.

APNOEA

It is stoppage of respiration. Apnoea can occur while a person is sleeping; this type of apnoea is known as *sleep apnoea*. Other causes of apnoea include deglutition apnoea, Bezold – Jarish reflex, etc.

CHEYNE – STOKES RESPIRATION

It is the pattern of breathing in which the tidal volume increases then deceases in a regular series of cycles that are repeated over and over. This type of respiration may occur in normal individuals, e.g., hypoxia at high altitude, but more often seen in patients suffering from neurologic and / or circulatory disorders.

In patients with neurologic factors, there is hyperventilation, though the arterial PCO_2 is subnormal and it is not responsible for this, since arterial PO_2 is normal.

In patients with heart disease, this impairs the circulation time considerably. There is a definitive lag between the time well oxygenated blood leaves the pulmonary capillaries and reaches the chemoreceptors. Due to this the feed-back impulses that are necessary to effect the adaptation of ventilation with arterial gas levels on a moment-to-moment basis are not achieved. Thus, there is a successively increasing and decreasing tidal volumes of cheyne - stokes respiration.

DYSPNOEA

Dyspnoea means difficulty in breathing. It appears at rest while a considerable fraction of the breathing reserve is still intact.

It is not always a sign of disease. It occurs in healthy individuals also. When pulmonary ventilation exceeds 4 times the resting minute volume the level of ventilation is called dyspnoea point.

It may be due to increased work of breathing or due to altered discharge from airway receptors, lung receptors, or respiratory muscle proprioceptors.

In left ventricular failure the lungs are congested and, therefore, the patient may feel dyspnoeic. But this dyspnoea is worse on lying down; the patient feels much better on sitting or standing up. This type of postural dyspnoea is called *orthopnoea*.

CYANOSIS

It is the bluish discolouration of skin due to the presence of more than 5 g deoxigenated haemoglobin / 100 ml of blood in small blood vessels of the skin or mucous membranes.

This is because deoxygenated Hb is bluish in colour while oxygenated Hb is reddish. The common sites are lips, nails, ear lobes, cheeks and mucous membranes of the oral cavity.

Central cyanosis

Excess of deoxygenated Hb in small vessels may be there because all arterial blood in the body is poorly oxygenated.

It is called so because the underlying cause is at a level proximal to or close to that from where oxygenated blood is circulated to the whole body.

Peripheral cyanosis

It is due to stasis of blood in skin capillaries. It may be due to cutaneous vasoconstriction due to the exposure to cold or in circulatory shock. Due to poor blood flow, more O_2 is extracted to meet the metabolic needs of tissues from the blood flowing through capillaries.

ASPHYXIA

It is the acute effect produced by hypoxia and hypercapnia together.

Effects of low atmospheric pressure

The low atmospheric pressure exists / increases as we ascend the high altitude. The effects produced due to this are :

Hyperventilation : It starts due to hypoxic hypoxia which stimulates the carotid body chemoreceptors which increases the ventilation.

Work capacity : It is decreased due to acute effect of high altitude.

2, 3 – DPG conc. : Increases within hours of exposure to high altitude or hypoxia.

Acidity : Increases pH in the RBC due to increase in deoxy Hb which binds more H^+ ions.

Effects of high atmospheric pressure

Various effects produced are :

Oxygen supply and oxygen toxicity : Since at high pressure like under water, there is oxygen deficiency which leads to hypoxia. In order to prevent this a mixture of gases is provided. But in this high saturation of Hb with O_2 lead to.

Impair uptake of Co_2 from tissues : High Po_2 in tissues will lead to generation of free radicals which oxidizes the pufa or cell membranes and some intracellular enzymes.

This can be prevented by giving the person a gas mixture with low O_2 conc. To breathe instead of normal air.

1. Carbon dioxide build-up due to less removal and ↑ O_2 uptake.
2. N_2 toxicity

At normal ATM pressure N_2 is inert but at high ATM. Pressure, it dissolves gradually into body fluids and fats. It has a depressant action on the nervous system.

It causes main damage by forming air bubbles in the tissues and fat components of body when the person ascends rapidly.

ACCLIMATIZATION

These are the changes that occur in an individual when he ascends a high attitude which help him to live better. It involves :

1. Reduce the pressure drop during transfer.
2. Increased the O_2 carrying capacity of blood, and
3. Improve the ability of the tissues to utilise O_2.

This helps in adapting the body so that the highlander is comfortable and his work capacity is equal to lowlander.

Mountain Sickness

These are the adverse effects which occur when a person ascends a high altitude :

High altitude pulmonary oedema : Due to pulmonary vascular hypertension which is due to hypoxia and high cardiac output.

Cerebral oedema : Due to response of cerebral blood vessels to hypoxia.

Chronic mountain sickness : It develops slowly due to an aberration in normal respiratory physiological responses to high altitude. It involves :

1. Increased haemoglobin level which increases viscosity of blood leading to poor oxygenation which causes mental fatigue and headache.
2. Wide spread vasoconstriction due to hypoxia.

ARTIFICIAL RESPIRATION

Respiratory arrest may occur as a result of drowning, poisoning, suffocation, electrocution, myocardial infarction. To restore the oxygen supply of body and to prevent death, artificial respiration is given. It involves :

Mouth-to-mouth method

It is the simplest method. In this while maintaining the head tilt to keep the tongue out of way, air is blown into the victim's chest through an air tight mouth-to-mouth contact. While doing this the nostrile of victim are kept closed. After a reasonable amount of air has blown in, the rescuer moves his mouth from victim's mouth and watches the chest to deflate itself. The procedure is repeated 12-20 times / minute.

CAISSON'S DISEASE

Caisson is a chamber in which the men dig under water tunnel. The high atmospheric pressure inside this prevents entry of water.

Caisson's disease is due to increased PN_2 in the blood of the person whose body is exposed to high atmospheric pressure. N_2 produce nitrogen narcosis due to high PN_2. The characteristic features of this disease are :

1. Euphoria.

2. Impaired mental functions.
3. Alcoholic intoxication symptoms.

Treatment

The subject should come to the surface slowly and if nitrogen narcosis occurs it is prevented by breathing O_2- Helium mixture, instead of N_2.

12
THE EXCRETORY SYSTEM

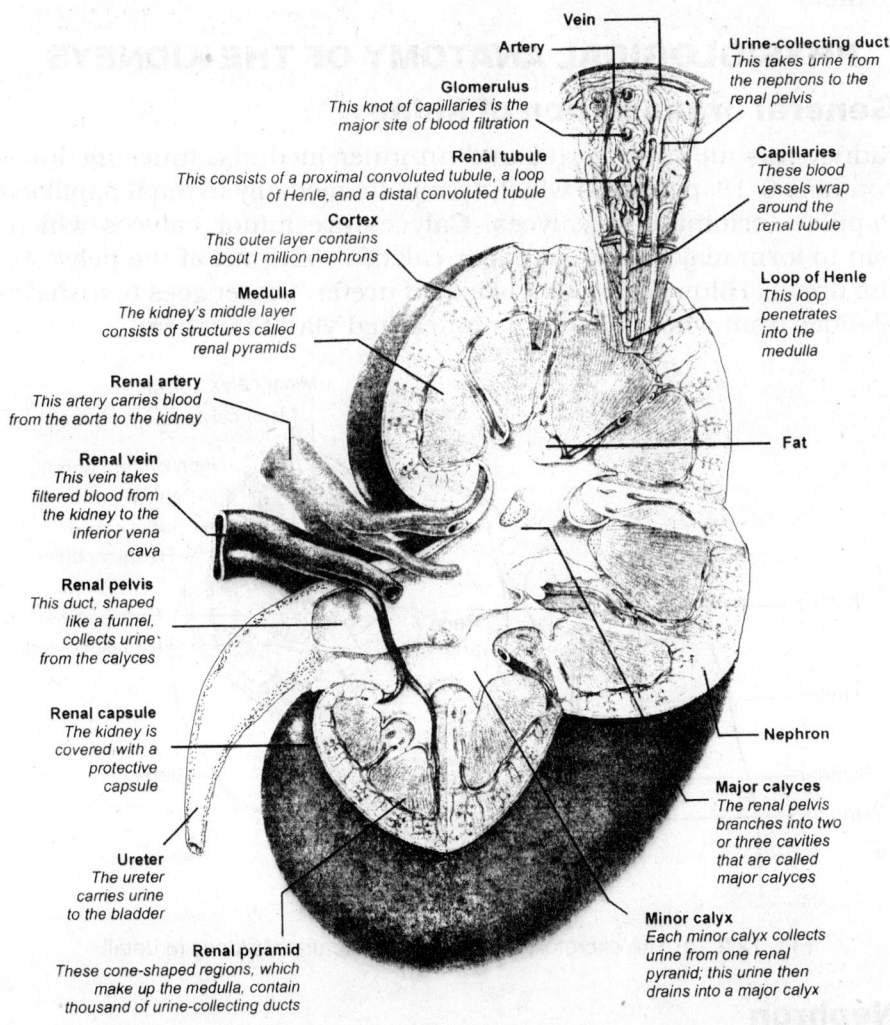

Fig. 12.1 Kidney.

KIDNEYS

Kidneys perform an important function to rid the body of waste material that are either ingested or produced by metabolism.

MICTURITION

It is the process by which the urinary bladder empties when filled.

MECHANISM OF FORMATION OF URINE

The nephrons of the kidneys clear the blood of certain substances. Substances which need to be excreated are removed by glomerular filtration and secretion from the tubules leading to formation of urine.

PHYSIOLOGICAL ANATOMY OF THE KIDNEYS

General organization of kidney

Kidney has an outer cortex and an inner medulla. Inner medulla contains 9-18 pyramids which terminate medially to renal papillae. Papillae terminate in calyces. Calyces are minor calyces which join to form major calyces; major calyces come out of the pelvis to the ureter. Hilus is the point of exit of ureter. Ureter goes to urinary bladder from where bladder is evacuated via the urthera.

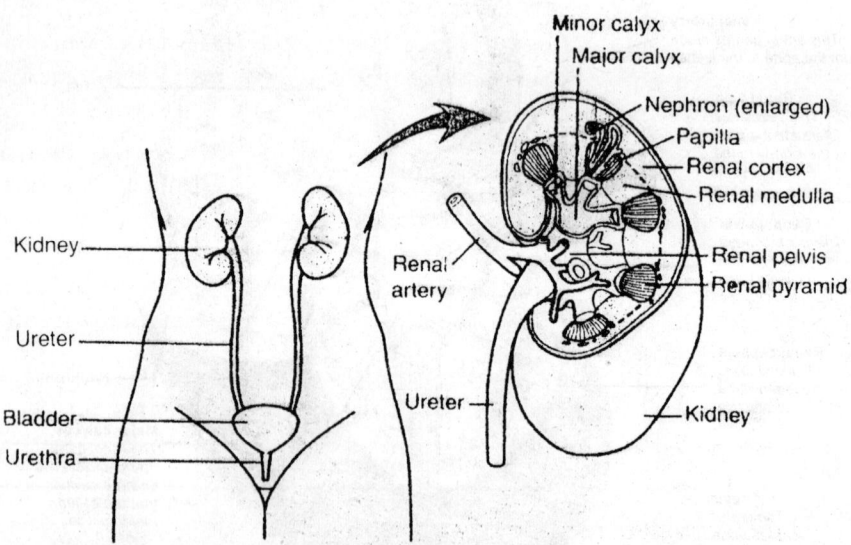

Fig. 12.2 (a) The excretory system. (b) Structure of kidney in detail.

Nephron

Each kidney contains about one million of nephrons. Nephrons are the functional unit of the kidney. Nephron consists of following parts :

1. Bowman's capsule
2. Glomerulus
3. Proximal convoluted tubule
4. Loop of henle
5. Distal convoluted tubule
6. Collecting tubules.

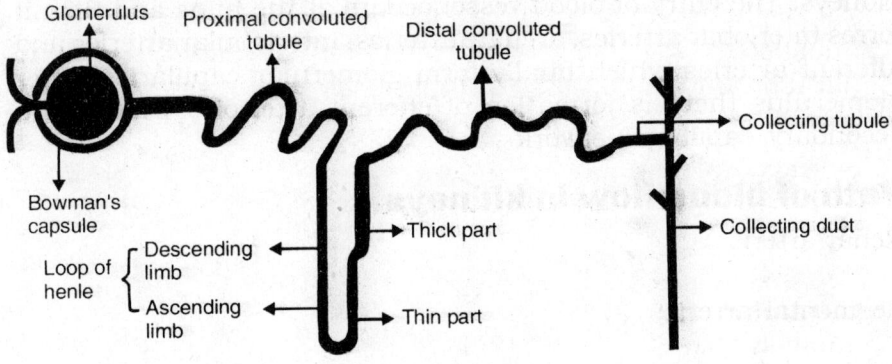

Fig. 12.3 Nephron.

Types of Nephrons : Depending upon the depth of nephrons within the kidneys, the nephrons have been divided into two groups — Cortical nephrons and juxta-medullary nephrons.

Cortical nephrons are in the larger amount as compared to juxta-medullary nephrons. On one side the cortical nephrons have glomeruli located in the outer cortex, the other side the juxta-medullary nephrons lie deep in the renal cortex. Blood supply of cortical nephron is from particular capillary plexus as compared to vasa recta supplying juxta-medullary nephrons.

Difference between the 2 types of Nephrons :

	Juxta-medullary	Cortical
1. Number	Less ~ 15%	More ~ 85%
2. Glomeruli size and location	Larger. At the corticomedullary junction	Smaller. In renal contex
3. Looks of Henle	Longer	Shorter
4. Vascular supply of loop of henle	Vasa recta	Peritubullar capillary plexus
5. Urine concentrating power	More	Less

Renal blood flow shows phenomenon of auto regulation, i.e., if the vascular resistance decreases there is decrease in perfusion pressure leading to decreased blood flow. Between 90-220 mmHg the renal blood flow shows autoregulatory phenomena despite change in arterial blood pressure.

BLOOD FLOW TO THE KIDNEY

Twenty-two percent of cardiac output is the blood flow to the two kidneys. The entry of blood vessel occurs at the hilus and then it forms interlobar arteries, arcuate arteries, interlobular arteries and afferent arteries which finally form glomerular capillaries. After glomerulus there is formation of efferent arterioles which form secondary capillary network.

Path of blood flow in kidneys

Renal artery
↓
Segmental arteries
↓
Interlobar arteries
↓
Arcuate arteries
↓
Interlobular arteries
↓
Afferent arterioles
↓
Glomerular capillaries
↓
Efferent arterioles
↓
Peritubular capillaries
↓
Interlobular veins
↓
Arcuate veins
↓
Renal vein

Some peculiarities of Renal Blood Flow

1. Presence of munerous tufts of capillaries called the glomeruli.
2. Glomerular capillaries have a much higher blood pressure (45 mmHg) than in the systemic capillaries (25 mmHg).
3. Portal system.

4. Glomerular capillaries are the only capillaries in the body which drain into arterioles.

URINE FORMATION

Urine formation occurs due to glomerular filtration, tubular secretion and tubular reabsorption.

Glomerular filteration

Glomerular capillaries are relatively impermeable to proteins, therefore, the filtered fluid is protein free and devoid of cellular elements like R.B.Cs. Since the calcium and plasma fatty acids are bound to the proteins, therefore, the filtrate is devoid of these contents. Otherwise, the osmolality and electrical conductivity are same as the concentration of other constituents of the glomerular filtrate, including salt and organic matters are similar to the concentration in the plasma.

Glomerular filteration rate : It refers to the volume of glomerular filterate formed each minute by all the nephrons in both the kidneys. G.F.R. is about 20% of the renal plasma flow.

G.F.R. = Filteration fraction x renal plasm flow

Normal value – 125 ml / min.

G.F.R. changes with advancing age, hydrostatic pressure in the Bowmans capsule, hydrostatic pressure in glomerular capillaries, plasma protein concentration, capillary bed size.

This is because :

G.F.R. = Kf x Net filteration pressure

Kf — Filteration coefficient

Net filteration pressure = $(P_G - P_B - K_G + K_B)$

P_G — Hydrostatic pressure in glomerular capillaries

P_B — Hydrostatic pressure in Bowman's capsule.

K_G — Colloid osmotic pressure of glomerular capillary plasma proteins.

K_B — Colloid osmotic pressure of proteins in the Bowman's capsule.

Tubuloglomerular feedback : Decrease in the flow of fluid through ascending limb of the loop of henle and first part of distal convoluted tubule causes increase in G.F.R. and *vice versa*. It is a macula densa feedback mechanism for auto regulation of glomerular hydrostatic pressure and glomerular filteration rate during change in renal arterial pressure.

Tubular secretion

It is the secretion of certain substances from the peritubular capillaries into the tubular lumen.

Tubular reabsorption

It is the active transport of solutes and passive absorption of water from tubular lumen to the peritubular capillaries.

> **Transport maximum :** It refers to the maximal amount of solute that can be reabsorbed. It is due to saturation of the specific transport systems.
>
> The glucose transport system in the proximal tubule is a good example to explain the transport maximum. Normally there is no excretion of glucose in the urine since all the glucose is reabsorbed. However, when the filtered load exceeds the tubular ability to reabsorb urinary excretion occurs.
>
> Transport maximum of certain substances is given below :
>
> Glucose – 320 mg / min
>
> Plasma protein – 30 mg / min
>
> Urate – 16 mg / min

MICTURITION REFLEX

Micturition reflex is a single cycle of following steps :

Basal tone of the bladder
↓
Progressive and rapid increase of pressure
↓
Sustained increase of pressure
↓
Emptying of the bladder
↓
Return of the pressure to the basal tone of the bladder

RENAL FUNCTIONS

Kidney plays a lot of functions which are as follows :

1. To rid the body of waste material that are either ingested or produced by metabolism.
2. Regulation of water and electrolyte balances.
3. Acid-base regulation.
4. Endocrinal functions :

- Renin
- Renal erythropoietic factor
5. Gluconeogenesis
6. Regulation of arterial pressure.
7. Body fluid osmolality and electrolyte concentration regulation.
8. Maintain the constancy of body internal environment.

JUXTA GLOMERULAR APPARATUS

Specialised tubular and vascular cells located at the vascular pole (where afferent and efferent arterioles enter and leave the glomerulus).

These specialised cells are :
1. Juxtaglomerular cells
2. Macula densa cells
3. Mesangial cells

Juxtaglomerular cells

Juxtaglomerular cells release a proteolytic enzyme called renin. This renin plays an important role in renin angiotensin system. This angiotensin is a generalized arteriolar constrictor and raises both systolic and diastolic blood pressure and also causes contraction of mesangial cells which in turn decreases G.F.R.

Renin angiotensin system is as follows :

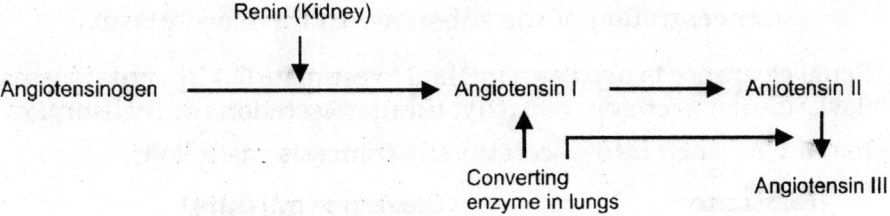

Angiotensin II causes vasoconstriction and renal retention of salt and water.

Macula densa cells

These detect decrease in Nacl load and cause increase in renin release.

Mesangial cells

These are found between capillary loops of Juxta glomerular apparatus. They play role in regulation of the glomerular filtration.

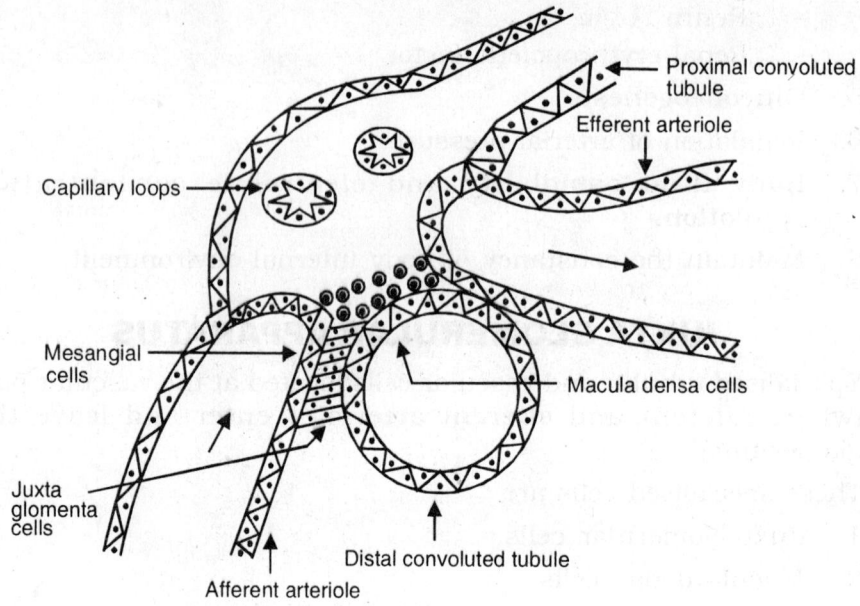

Fig. 12.4 Juxta glomerular apparatus.

CLEARANCE

Renal clearance of a substance is the volume of plasma that is completely cleared of the substance by the kidneys per unit time.

$$= \frac{\text{Renal clearance of a given substance is the ratio of renal excretion rate of the substance}}{\text{Concentration of the substance in the blood plasma}}$$

Renal clearance is used as a method to estimate G.F.R., renal plasma flow, tubular secretory capacity, tubular secretions or reabsorption.

Renal clearance rate of certain substances is as follows :

	Substance	Clearance (ml/min)
1.	Glucose	0.0
2.	Sodium	0.9
3.	Chloride	1.40
4.	Creatinine	140.0

RENAL TRANSPORT MECHANISM

As the filtrate passes along the proximal convoluted tubule all the protein, amino acids and glucose contained in the fluid are reabsorbed.

The amino acids and glucose are sodium gradient linked across the luminal membrane.

The driving force for their uptake is provided by the sodium pump of the basalateral membrane.

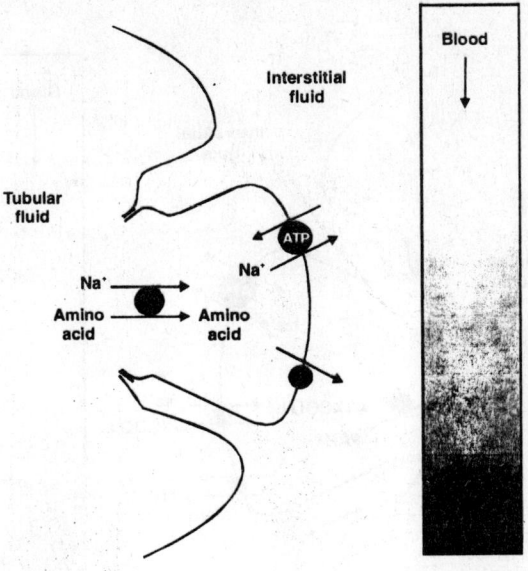

Fig. 12.5 Reabsorption of amino acids in proximal tubules.

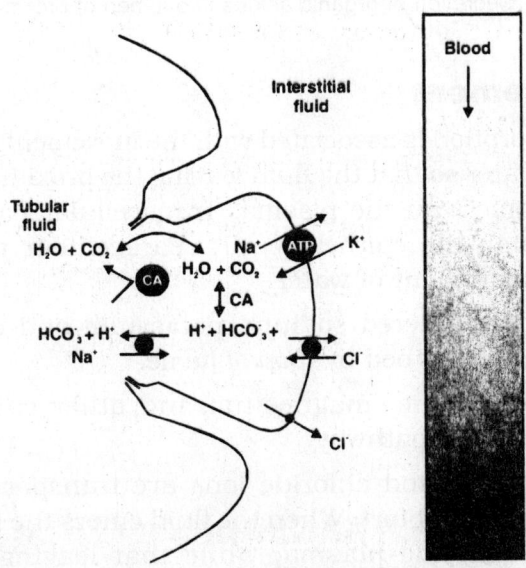

Fig. 12.6 Bicarbonate reabsorption in proximal tubule.

Almost all essential organic constituents in the tubular fluid are reabsorbed in the first half of tubule. Sodium absorption in the second half of proximal tubule is coupled to chloride.

Secretions in proximal convoluted tubules — Secretion of some organic anions and cations occurs in the tubular fluid.

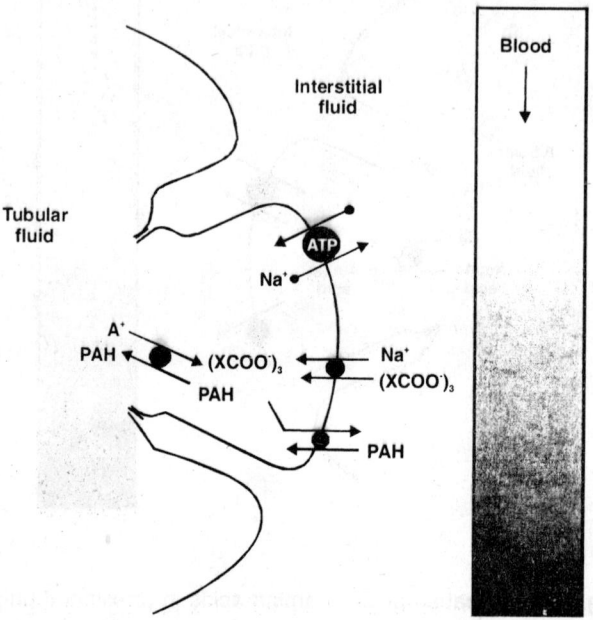

Fig. 12.7 Secretion of organic anions into lumen of proximal tubule.

Water movement

The solute absorption is associated with the movement of an osmotic equivalent of water so that the fluid leaving the proximal convoluted tubule is isotonic with the plasma. Transcellular pathway is the pathway through the epithelial cells. Paracellular pathway also contribute to movement of water.

About 20% of the filtered sodium, potassium and chloride ions with water are reabsorbed by *loop of henle.*

Absorption of calcium, magnesium and other cations occurs through paracellular pathway.

Sodium, potassium and chloride ions are transported from the tubular fluid by a symptort. When the fluid enters the loop of henle, it is isotonic with the plasma, while that leaving the loop is hypotonic due to tubular reabsorption of various ions.

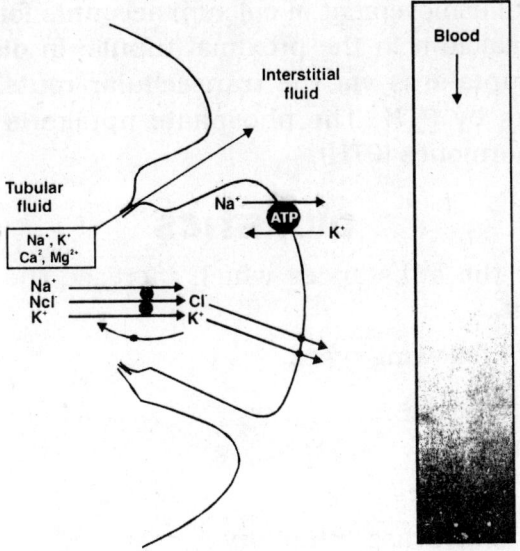

Fig. 12.8 Uptake of Na+ and Cl- in thick ascending limb of loop of henle.

In the *first part of the distal tubule* the dilution of tubular fluid continues.

Now comes the *second part of distal tubule* and the collecting duct, it contains P cells and intercalated cells. The sodium and water absorption occurs by P cell. Secretion of potassium is also by P cells. The secretion of hydrogen ions occurs by intercalated cells.

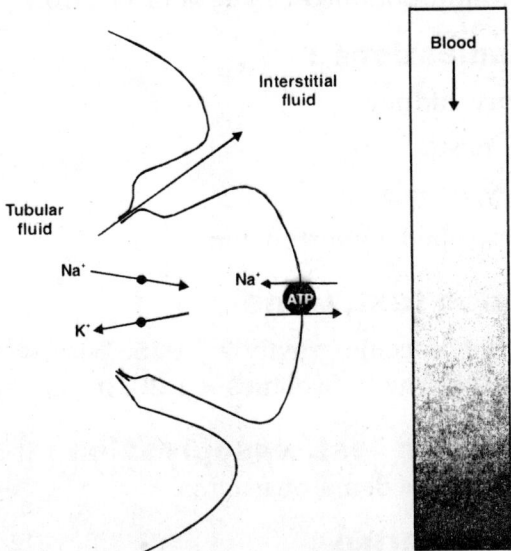

Fig. 12.9 Secretion of potassium ions in distal tubule and collecting duct.

The transcellular movement of calcium accounts for about a third of uptake of calcium in the proximal tubule; in distal tubule all the calcium uptake is via the transcellular route. The calcium uptake occurs by PTH. The phosphate uptake is decreased by parathyroid hormones (PTH).

DIURETICS

Diuretics are the substances which increase the rate of urine volume output.

Diuretes are of following types :

1. Osmotic diuretics
2. Loop diuretics
3. Thiazide diuretics
4. Carbonic anhydrase inhibitory
5. Sodium channel blockers
6. Potassium sparing diuretics

KIDNEY FUNCTION TESTS

Renal Biopsy

Renal Biopsy should be preceded by confirmation that no renal infection is present.

Examination includes histology (stained by H&E, PAS, Silver and other stains), immunofluorescence, and electron microscopy.

Contraindications :

1. Solitary kidney
2. Large cyst
3. Kidney neoplasm
4. Uncontrolled hypertension

Concentration test, urine

Normal urine has specific gravity ≥ 1.025. With decreased kidney functions, specific gravity becomes < 1.20, it may approach 1.0.

Concentration test, vasopression : It can be used in the presence of oedema or ascites.

Urea nitrogen (BUN)

It is helpful in the diagnosis of renal insufficiency. A low BUN of

6-8 mg/dl is frequently associated with states of over-hydration. BUN 10-20 mg/dl indicates normal glomerular functions. BUN of 50-150 mg/dl indicates seriously, impaired function.

Creatine

Serum creatine is a more specific and sensitive indicator of renal disease as compared to BUN.

Serum creatine is increased in :

1. Muscle disease.
2. Intake of roast meat.
3. Prerenal and postrenal Azotemias.

Serum creatine decreases in pregnancy.

Blood urea nitrogen (BUN) / creatine ratio

Normal range for a healthy person on normal diet — 12-20.

It is used to differentiate pre and postrenal azotemia from renal azotemia.

Glomerular filteration rate (G.F.R.)

The creatinine clearance test, particularly serial measure-ment, is the most reliable test for renal function. Serum creatinine level can be used to calculate clearance.

Interpretation — G.F.R. begins to decrease after age of 40.

Usually good correlation is seen between urine concentration test and G.F.R. A normal G.F.R. associated with impaired concentrating ability may be found in the sickle cell anaemia, diabetes insipidus, and various acquired disorders like hypercalciuria.

Normal clearance — 1.73 ml/minute/sq cm of body surface area.

Urine osmolality

Urine osmolality measurement during water restriction is an accurate and sensitive test of decreased renal function.

Normal — Concentration is > 800 mosm/kg

Severe impairment — < 400 mosm/kg

Moderate impairment — 400-600 mosm/kg

Mild impairment — 600-800 mosm/kg.

Split renal function test

The affected kidney shows decreased urine volume and sodium excretion and decreased urine concentration of creatinine, inulin.

Phenol sulfon phalein (PSP) excretion test

It can detect mild to moderate decrease in renal function.

Normal : > 25% in urine in 15 min.

        55-75% in 2 hrs.

Acute glomerulonephritis is suspected in cases where PSP is normal with increased BUN and serum creatine and decreased GFR.

13

THE NERVOUS SYSTEM

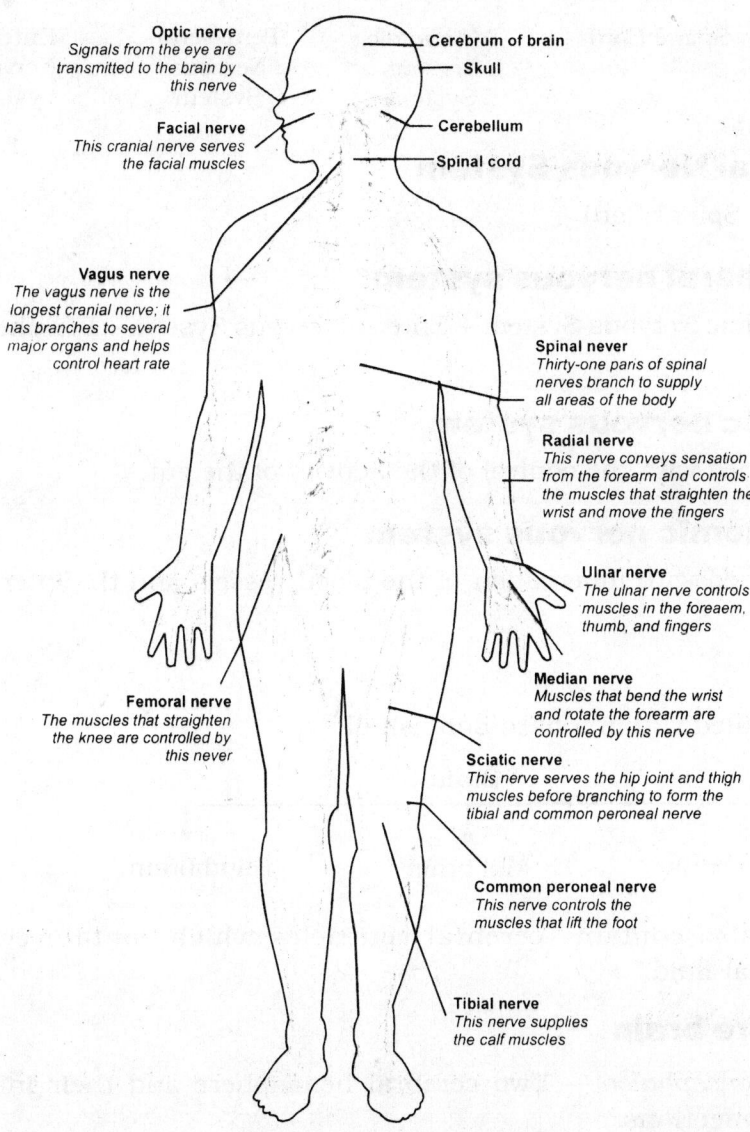

Fig. 13.1 Nervous system.

INTRODUCTION

Integration of sensory information occurs at all levels of nervous system. This leads to subsequent and appropriate motor responses, beginning in the spinal cord extending to cerebrum, where most of the complicated responses are controlled.

Nervous system is divided into following parts :

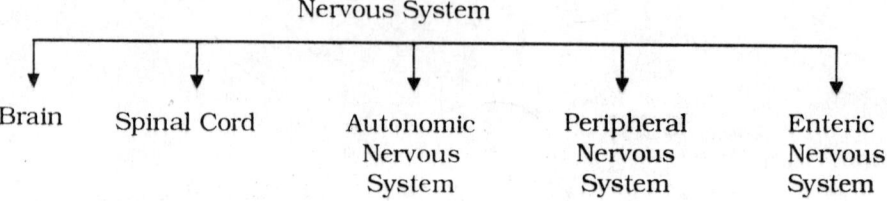

Central Nervous System

Brain + Spinal Cord.

Peripheral nervous system

Autonomic Nervous System + Enteric Nervous System + Peripheral nerves

Enteric nervous system

Concerned with the control of the activity of the gut.

Autonomic nervous system

Concerned with innervation of the blood vessels and the internal organs.

Brain

It is located within a hard bony skull

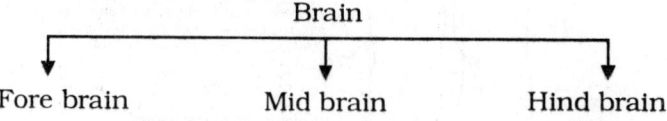

Brain also contains cerebral ventricles which contain cerebrospinal fluid.

Fore brain

Telencephalon — Two cerebral hemisphere and their interconnections.

Diencephalon — Thalamus and hypothalamus.

Mid brain
1. Cerebral peduncle
2. Tectum

Hind brain
1. Pons
2. Medulla oblongata
3. Cerebellum

Spinal cord
1. *Lies outside the skull.* It is a long cylindrical structure.
2. An anterior fissure known as anterior median fissure.
3. A posterior fissure known as posterior median fissure.
4. Grey matter contains nerve cells.
5. Posterior horn receives the fibres of posterior roots which are purely sensory.
6. Anterior horn contain cells bodies of α, and ren shaw motor neurons and nerve fibres which are purely motor.
6. Surrounding the grey matter is white matter consisting of ascending and descending axous.

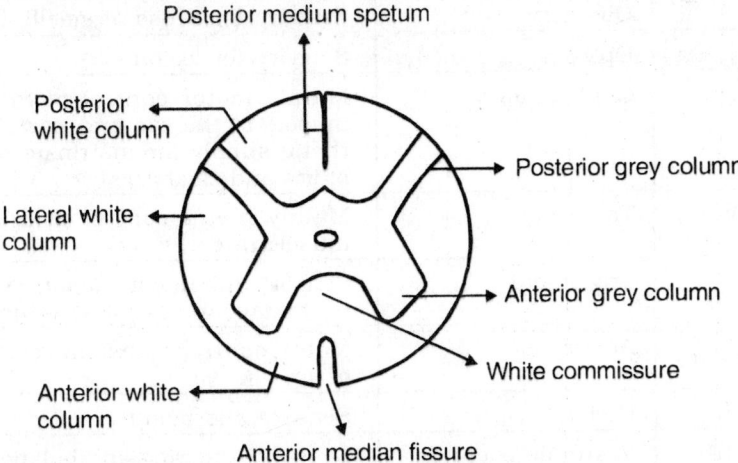

Fig. 13.2 Transverse section of spinal cord showing arrangement of white and grey matter.

PERIPHERAL NERVOUS SYSTEM

It is divided as follows :
1. Autonomic nervous system

(a) Sympathetic nervous system
(b) Parasympathetic nervous system
2. Periperal nerves and enteric nerves
   (a) Spinal nerves
   (b) Cranial nerves

Spinal nerves — 31 pair

(i)   Cervical   —   8
(ii) Thoracic   —   12
(iii) Lumbar   —   5
(iv) Sacral   —   5
(v)   Coccygeal —   1

Cranial nerves — 12 pairs

Types :
(i)   Sensory
(ii) Motor
(iii) Mixed

Cranial nerves — (OOOTTAFAGVAH)

Number	Name	Chief function
I	Olfactory	Sensory for sense of smell
II	Optic	Sensory for vision
III	Oculomotor	Mainly motor control of extrinsic muscle of the eye and parasympathetic supply for instrinsic muscle of iris and ciliary body
IV	Trochlear	Mainly motor control of extrinsic muscle of eye
V	Trigeminal	Sensory and motor — motor control of the jaw and facial sensation
VI	Abducens	Motor control of extrinsic muscle of eye
VII	Facial	Sensory and motor
VIII	Vestibulo-cochlear	Sensory – hearing and balance
IX	Glossopharyngeal	Sensory and motor control of swallowing
X	Vagus	Major parasympathetic outflow to the chest and abdomen. Afferent inputs from the viscera
XI	Spinal accessory	Motor — neck muscles and larynx
XII	Hypoglossal	Motor to tongue

ACTION POTENTIAL PROPAGATION

After initiation of action potential it is transmitted along the entire length of an axon. When peak occurs the action potential is positive. During propagation of action potential two different zones are created in the nerve fibre — an active one and a resting zone. Finally leading to formation of a local circuit which links the active zone to the neighbouring resting zone.

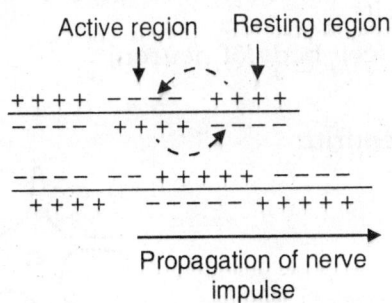

Propagation of nerve impulse

If the nerve is myelinated, current can only cross the axon membrane at the nodes of Ranvier. Thus, action potential is saltatory (jumping) type.

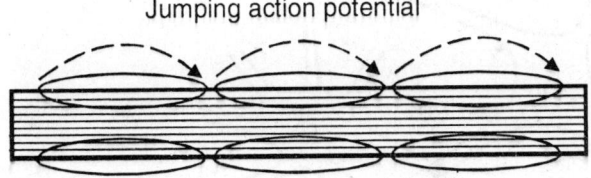

Jumping action potential

Larger the diameter of the nerve faster the conduction. Myelinated nerve fibres conduct faster as compared to non-myelinated nerve fibres.

Threshold

Action potential is generated when a neuron is activated by a stimulus of a certain minimum strength.

All or none law

With the stimuli above threshold each action potential has approximately same magnitude and duration.

Action potential

A short-lived increase in the permeability of the membrane to sodium ion causes action potential. This is due to opening of voltage-gated sodium channels. After some time sodium channels inactivate spontaneously. Voltage-gated sodium channel cannot reopen untill they reach resting membrane potential.

SYNAPSE

A specialized junction formed when an axon reaches its target cells.

Types

1. Axon with dendrite
2. Axon with soma (cell body of neuron)
3. Axon with axon
4. Dendrite with dendrite

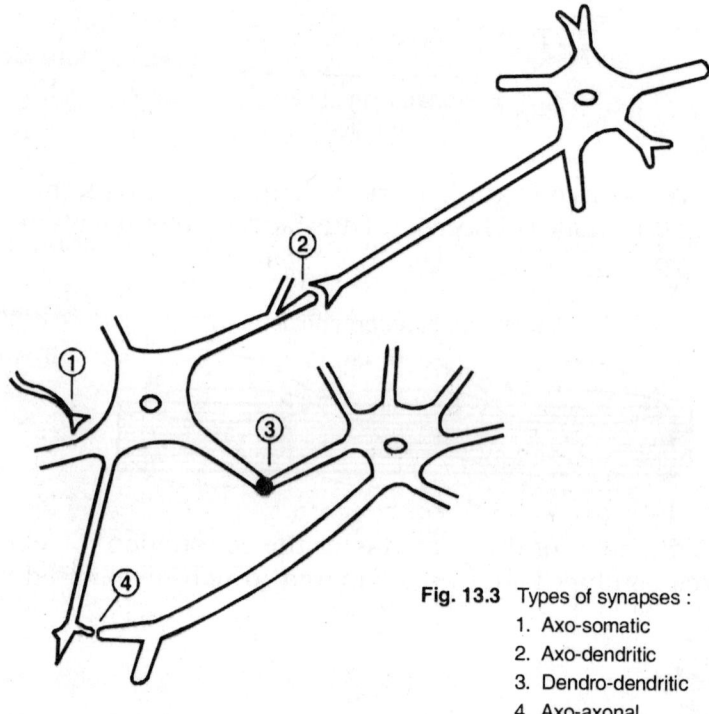

Fig. 13.3 Types of synapses :
1. Axo-somatic
2. Axo-dendritic
3. Dendro-dendritic
4. Axo-axonal

These synapses can be :

Chemical — Transmission of impulse by chemical mediator.

Electrical — Transmission is electrical.

Conjoint — Both chemical and electrical transmission.

Synapse

It is a junctin between a neuron and another neuron or some other tissue.

Excitatory : When the activity of the post synaptic cell increases.

Inhibitory : When the activity of the post synaptic cell decreases. It can be postsynaptic or presynaptic inhibition.

NEURO TRANSMITTERS

Two types of neuratransmitters are present :
1. Excitatory
2. Inhibitory

A given neuro transmitter may be excitatory in some location and inhibitory in others.

Neurotransmitters may also be classified on the basis of size :
1. Low molecular transmitters e.g. acetylcholine, amino acids, amines, nitric oxide.
2. Neuro peptides – composed of 3-40 amino acids.

RECEPTORS

It is a specialized sensory nerve ending which sends infor-mation to the CNS after undergoing depolarization.

Receptors can be : Skin senses receptors, visceral senses receptors, deep senses receptors, special senses receptors.

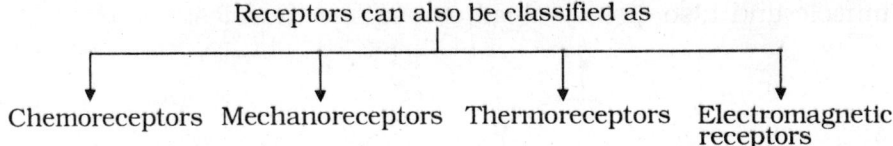

Chemoreceptors Mechanoreceptors Thermoreceptors Electromagnetic receptors

Skin contains receptors for touch, pain and temperature. Cutaneous receptors include Merkels discs, naked nerve endings, Pacinian corpuscles and Raffinis end organs.

Thermoreceptors can be for cold and warm. Pain receptors are known as nociceptors.

REFLEX

It is defined as automatic response to a stimusus.

Reflex arc includes at least two neurons — an afferent or sensory neuron and an efferent or motor neuron. Information about the environment is carried towards the CNS by afferent neuron while the transmission of impulse from CNS to an effector occurs by efferent neuron. Reflexes can be polysynaptic or monosynaptic. Polysynaptic reflexes includes those reflexes in which one or more, interneurons are present connecting afferent and efferent neurons, e.g., withdrawal reflexes. While those reflexes in which only one synapse is present between afferent and efferent neurons are known as monosynaptic reflexes, e.g., strech reflexes. The two kinds of reflexes differ from each other but they have some similarities like both of them are protective reflexes and involve reciprocal innervation.

The simplest reflexes are the monosynaptic strech reflexes such as the knee-jerk reflex.

Knee jerk reflex

Joints such as knee and ankle are extended and flexed by extensors and flexor muscles which act as antagonists. A sharp tap to patellar tendon stretches the quadriceps muscle. This stimulates afferent neurons. This inturn excites α–motor neurons supplying that muscle and causes its contraction.

Polysynaptic reflexes

Example is withdrawal reflex. The protective flexion is caused due to noxious stimuli. These reflexes possess at least one interneuron. Usually many muscle are involved through polysynaptic pathways which involve many spinal segments.

Stretch reflex

Stretching of a muscle suddenly causes excitation of spindles leading to contraction of larger skeletal muscle fibres of the same muscle and also closely allied synergistic muscles.

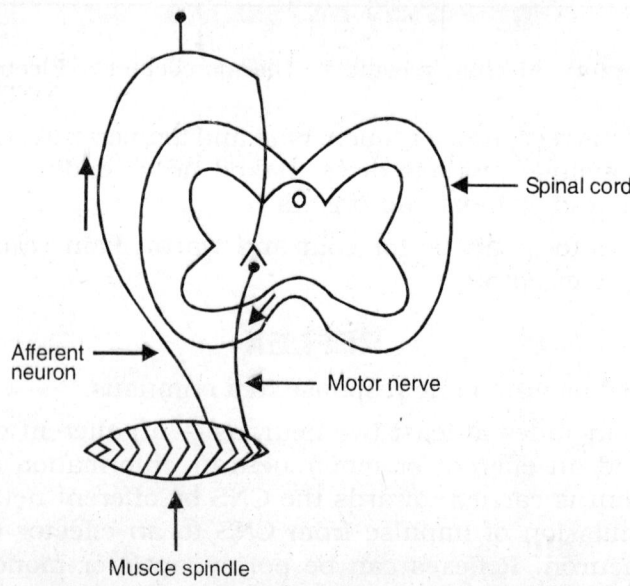

Fig. 13.4 Basic neuronal circuit of stretch reflex.

Factors controlling stretch reflex :
(a) Brain
  (i) Facilitatory reticular formation
  (ii) Vestibular nucleus
  (iii) Inhibitory reticular formation
(b) Anxiety
(c) Unexpected movements

*Stretch reflex inhibition can be reciprocal inhibition or inverse stretch reflex.

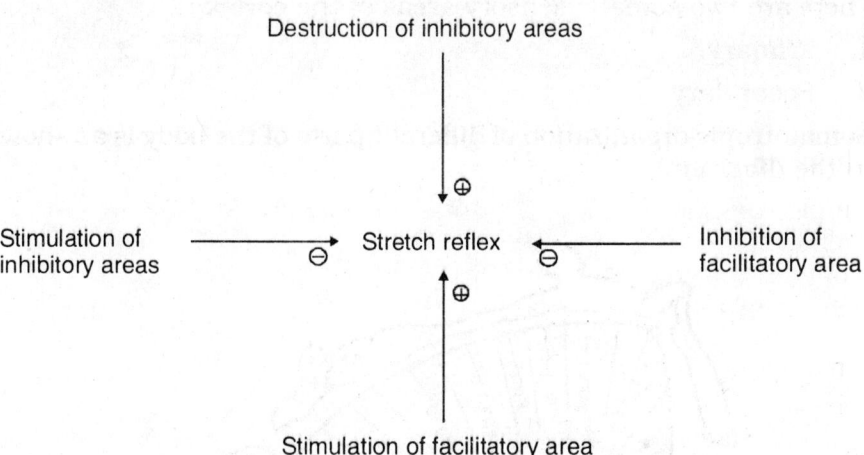

SENSORY PATHWAYS

Sensory system involves the cortex, the neural pathways and sensory receptors.

Sensory tracts

The ascending tracts, in spinal cord, from the peripheral receptors to the CNS. The tracts are divided into ventral, dorsal and lateral column.

Dorsal column :
1. Fasciculus gracilis.
2. Fasciculus cuneatus.

Ventral column : Ventral spinothalamic tract

Lateral column :
1. Lateral spinothalamic tract
2. Dorsal and ventral spinocerebellar tract

Fine touch, vibration, tactile sensations are conveyed by fasciculus gracilis and fasciculus cuneatus.

Uncontrolled kinesthetic sensations are passed by post-erior spinocerebellar tract and anterior spinocerebellar tract.

Lateral spinothalamic tracts convey pain and temprature.

Gross touch is conveyed by anterior spinothalamic tract.

Cortex

The cortex concerned with sensory function is known as somatosensory cortex.

There are two somatic sensory areas of the cortex :

1. Primary
2. Secondary

Somatotropic organization of different parts of the body is as shown in the diagram.

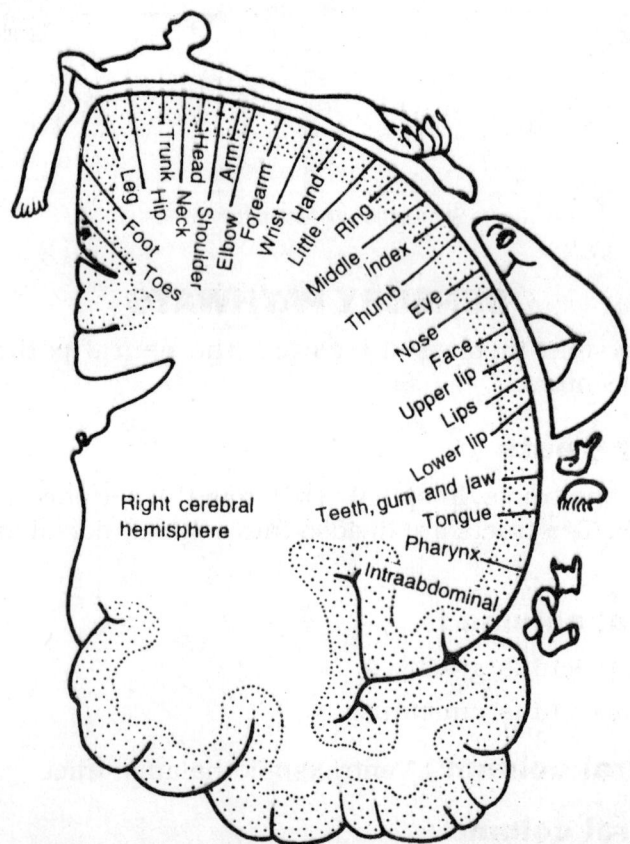

Fig. 13.5 Somatotropic organization of different body parts in somatosensory cortex.

Somatic sensation

1. Touch — pressure.
2. Proprioception — Sense of body position in space.
3. Kinesthetic — Sense of joint movement.
4. Temperature.
5. Pain.

> **Pain :** It is a sensation which draws attention of an individual as a whole. Pain can be superficial and deep.
>
> *Superficial pain* is sharp in character and well localized. It involves the skin and subcutaneous tissue.
>
> *Deep pain* : It involves muscles and hollow viscera and is dull and poorly localized. It is generally associated with nausea, vomiting.
>
> Pain receptors are known as nociceptors. Pain receptors are free nerve endings. They are widespread in superficial layers of skin as well as in certain internal tissues such as periosteum, arterial walls, joints etc.
>
> *Referred pain* : According to the principle of *dermatomal rule* the pain is reffered from a structure to another structure that developed from the same segment during the embryonic development.
>
> Example : Appendicitis pain is reffered to the umbilicus.

MOTOR PATHWAY

Motor system includes motor cortex, descending tracts.

Descending tracts

Pyramidal tracts, extrapyramidal tracts.

Pyramidal tracts

It includes corticobulbar and corticospinal tracts.

Extrapyramidal tracts

Areas other than pyramidal and cerebellar system but are involved in control of muscular movement and posture. It includes :

1. Medial longitudinal fasciculus
2. Tectospinal and tectobulbar tract
3. Vestibulospinal tract
4. Rubrospinal tract

5. Reticulospinal tract
   (Mnemonic — MTV **Red** **Ro**se)

Cortex

Representation of body in the motor cortex is as shown in the following diagram.

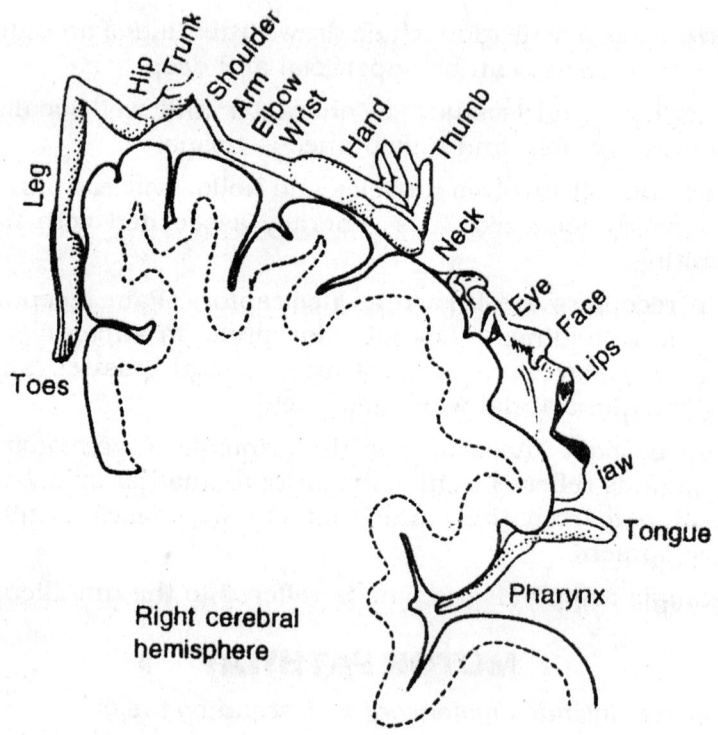

Fig. 13.6 Representation of body in motor cortex.

Functions of descending tracts

Pyramidal tracts :

1. Convey motor impulses to spinal cord for controlling the voluntary movements.
2. Voluntary control of muscles of larynx, pharynx, palate and upper and lower face.
3. Superficial reflexes.

Extrapyramidal tracts :

1. Control of posture, tone and equilibrium, eye movements.
2. Control complex movements of body and limb.

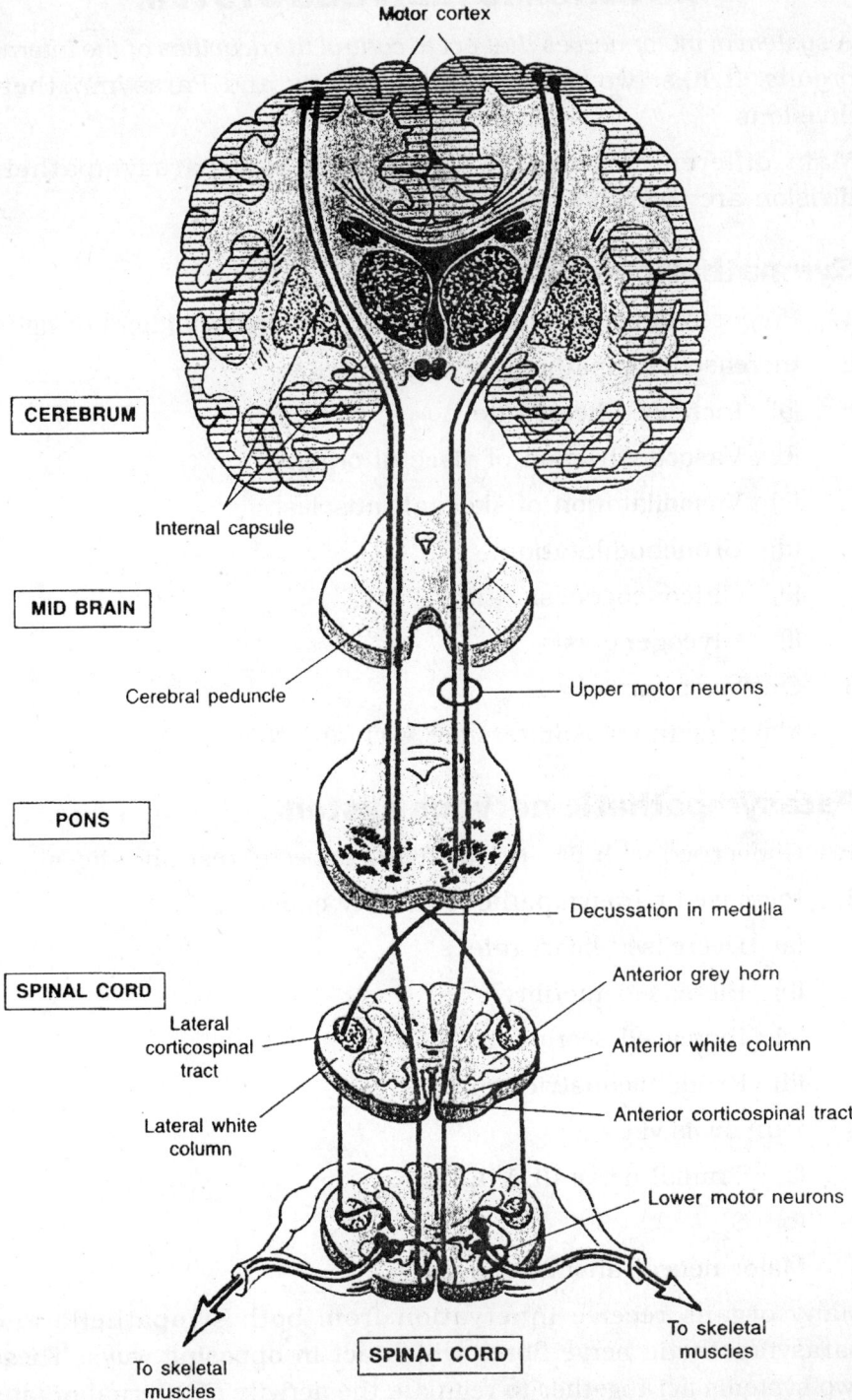

Fig. 13.7 Pyramidal pathways.

AUTONOMIC NERVOUS SYSTEM

A system of motor nerves that act to control the activities of the internal organs. It has two parts — Sympathetic and Parasympathetic divisions.

Main differences between sympathetic and parasympathetic division are given below:

Sympathetic nervous system

1. Prepares individual to cope with the emergency (flight or fight).
2. Increased sympathetic activity causes.
   (a) Increased heart rate.
   (b) Vasoconstriction of visceral organs.
   (c) Vasodilatation of skeletal muscles.
   (d) Bronchodilatation.
   (e) Gluconeogenesis and
   (f) Glycogenolysis
3. Outflow is via $T_1 \rightarrow L_3$
4. Major neurotransmitters are A-ch and NE

Parasympathetic nervous system

1. Concerned with day to day living aspects (rest and digest).
2. Increased parasympathetic activity cause :
   (a) Decreased heart rate
   (b) Increased motility
   (c) Increased secretions of GIT
   (d) Bronchoconstriction
3. Outflow is via —
   (a) Cranial nerve III, VII, IX, X
   (b) $S_{2,3,4}$
4. Major neurotransmitter is A-ch.

Many organs receive innervation from both sympathetic and parasympathetic nerve fibres which act in opposing ways. These two systems act together to regulate the activity of internal organs according to the needs of the body at a time. ANS is controlled by brain stem and hypothalamus.

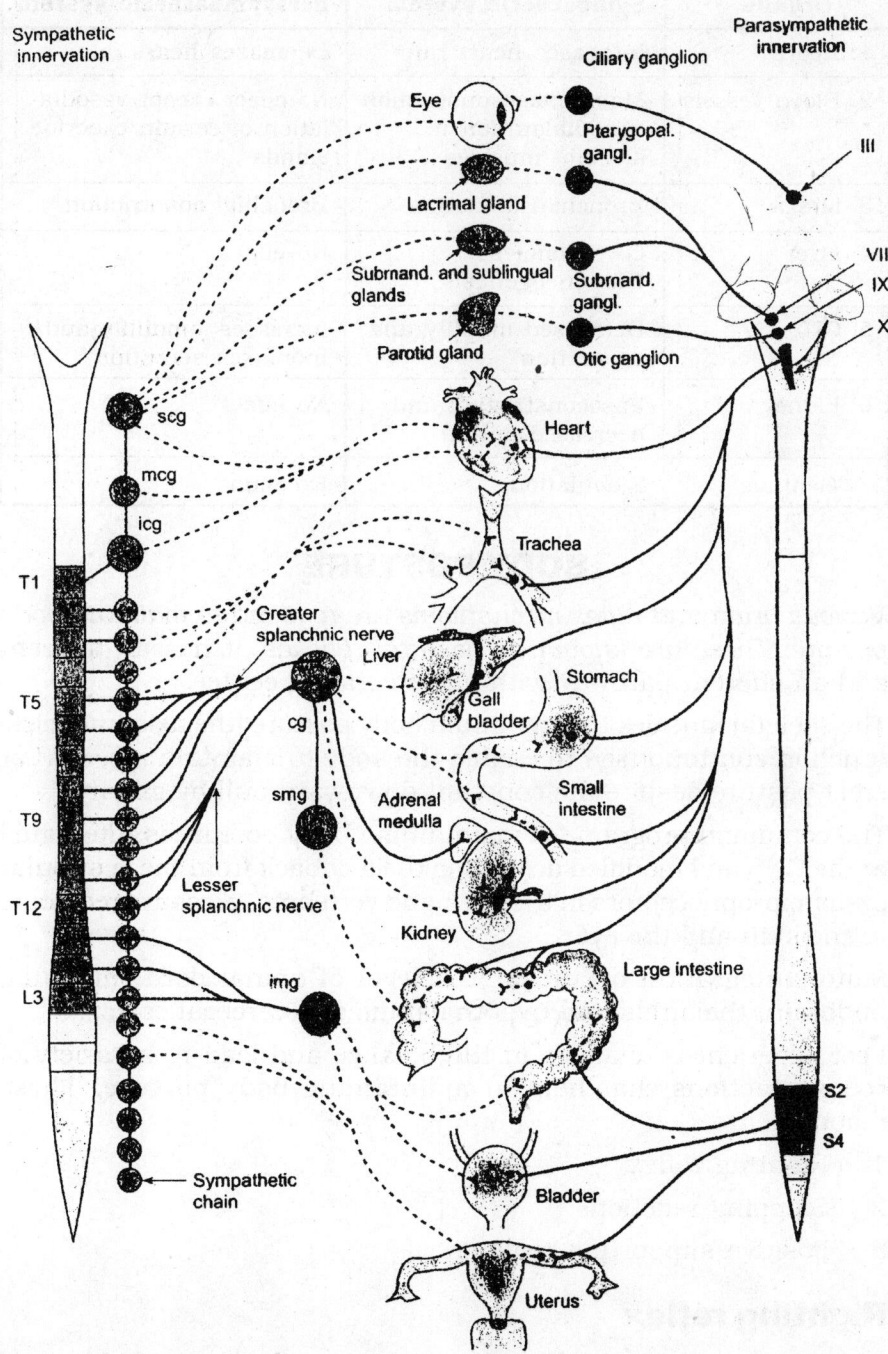

Fig. 13.8 The autonomic nervous system.

Major effects of ANS activities :

Organs	Sympathetic system	Parasympathetic system
1. Heart	Increases heart rate	Decreases heart rate
2. Blood vessels	Mainly vasoconstriction Vasodialatation in skeletal muscles	No effect except vasodialation of certain exocrine glands
3. Lungs	Bronchial dilatation	Bronchial constriction
4. Liver	Glycogenolysis, Gluconeogenesis	No effect
5. GIT	Decreased motility and secreation	Increases motility and increases secretion
6. Kidney	Vasoconstriction and decreased output	No effect
7. Genitals	Ejaculation	Erection

BODY POSTURE

Various brain and reflex mechanisms are required to maintain body posture. These are known as postural reflexes. It has an afferent and an efferent pathway with an integrating center.

The skeletal muscles that maintain body posture (the axial muscles) function continuously, to enable the body to maintain a seated or erect posture despite the constant downward pull by gravity.

The command program for maintaining body posture is integrated in the CNS and modified according the feedback from the vestibular system, proprioceptors in the neck and vertebrae, pressure receptors in the skin and the eyes.

Motor integration occurs at the level of spinal cord, medulla, midbrain, thalamus and hypothalamus and cerebral cortex.

Feet experiences changes in the balance and lead to a variety of reflex reactions that help in maintaining body posture. These reactions are :

1. Righting reflex
2. Stepping reactions
3. Positive supporting reaction

Righting reflex

A decerebrated animal placed on its side will move its limbs and head in an attempt to right itself. With the help of righting reflexes the midbrain animal can bring its head right way up and get the body into the erect position.

Positive supporting reaction

If the sole of feet of an animal, held in mid air, is pressed there will be reflex extension of the corresponding limb that will act to support the weight of the body.

Vestibular apparatus

It is a sensory organ which detects sensations of equilibrium. It is made up of bony tubes and chambers located inside temporal bone known as bony labyrinth. Inside this bony labyrinth resides membranous labyrinth (which is the functional unit).

Parts of vestibular apparatus (membranes labysinth):

1. Three semicircular canals
2. The otolith organ.

The semicircular canal : Three membranous canals namely horizontal, superior and inferior. Each is at right angle to the other. They contain endolymph.

The otolith organ : It consists of two sac-like swellings — the saccule and the utricle. Ductus endolymphaticus makes communication between the two sacs.

Both the saccule and the utricle contain specific receptors known as the crista and macula.

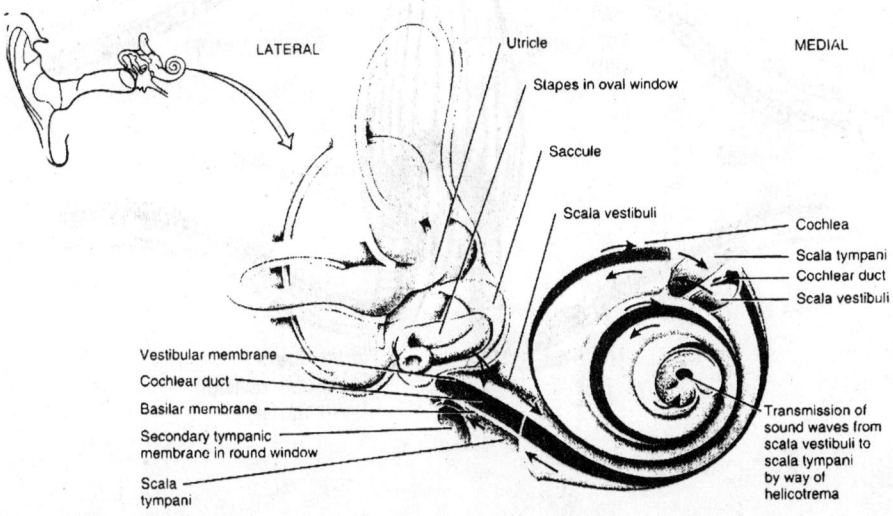

Fig. 13.9 The vestibular apparatus.

The crista and the macula are projecting ridge as shown in the figure. Hair cells which are tall columnar epithelium cover them and a firm gelatinous material called cupula is attached to the hair cells.

Functions :

1. They enable the erect position of the head and the normal posture of the body.
2. Helps in recognition of the position and movement of the head.
3. The otolith organs are stimulated by the gravity and the semicircular canals by rotational movements.

Disorders :

1. *Motion sickness* — Tendency of yawning; increased salivation, nausea, headache, pallor.
2. *Meniers disease* — Vertigo and tinnitus and bouts of hearing loss.

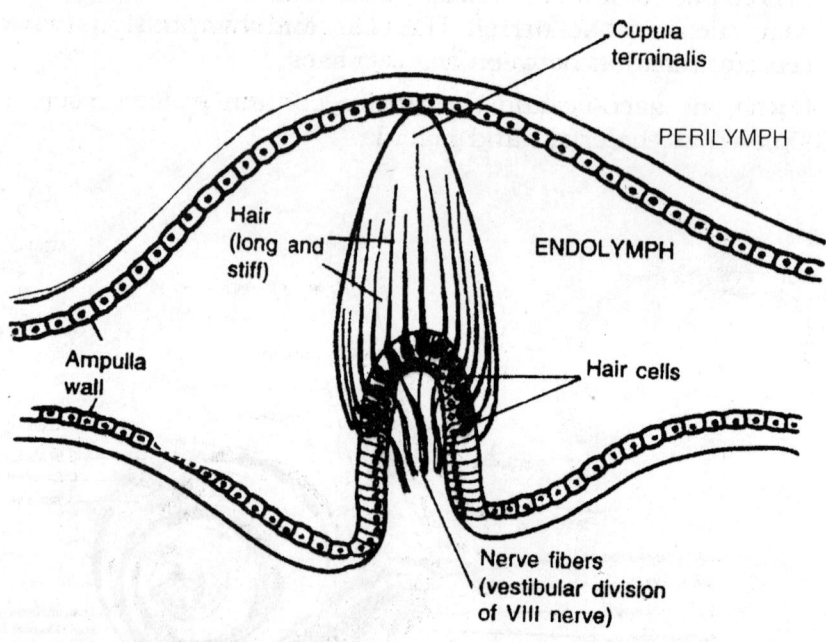

Fig. 13.10 Structure of crista.

The nervous system

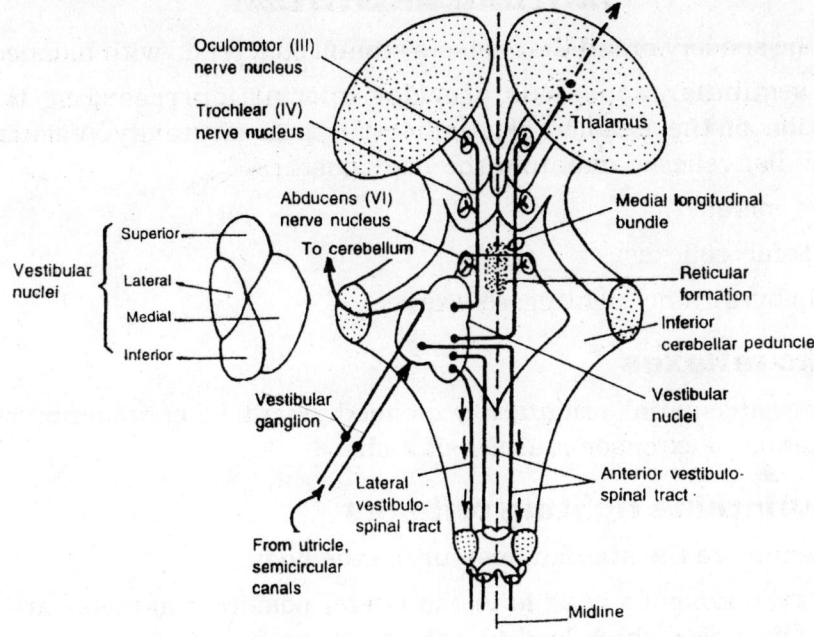

Fig. 13.11 Neural pathways from vestibular apparatus.

The nerve endings of crista and macula go to vestibular ganglion. The axons end in vestibular nuclei and then to cerebellum and III nerve. The fibres reach the opposite thalamus and thence the opposite temporal lobe.

Functioning of the vestibular apparatus

1. The saccule and utricle provide information about linear accelaration and head position.
2. The semicircular canals detect angular acceleration during rotation of the head along 3 perpendicular axes.

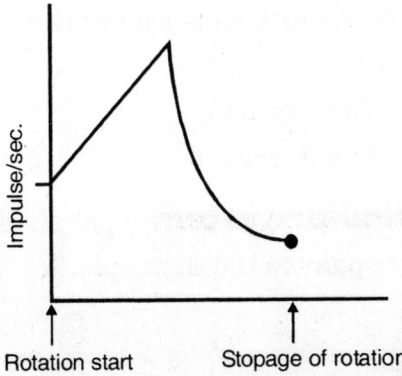

Fig.13.12 Response of hair cells when a semicircular canal is rotated and then stoped.

VESTIBULAR SYSTEM

It is the sensory organ that detects stimuli concerned with balance.

The vestibular apparatus provides information regarding the position of the head in relation to the pull of gravity. Various vestibular reflexes maintain the body posture.

These include :

1. Tonic reflexes
2. Labyrinthine righting reflexes

Tonic reflexes

Change in spatial orientation of head result in contraction or relaxation of extensor muscles of limbs.

Labyrinthine righting reflexes

These restore the standing posture of the body.

When the animal's head is in the lateral position, impulses arise in the saccules which lead to righting of the head.

Neck reflexes

Various proprioceptors in the neek and vertebral column provide information about head and body position in relation to each other.

Visual information

Supplementing action of retinal receptors is present. They supplement information from semicircular canals of the vestibular system.

RETICULAR FORMATION

It is an essential part of brain composed of parts of brain stem which are characterized by an interlacing network of fiber bundle.

Reticular formation :

1. Ascending reticular system.
2. Descending reticular system.

Ascending reticular system

It extend from lower pons to the thalamus.

Functions :

1. Perception
2. Wakefulness and alertness.

Descending reticular system

Descend to spinal cord.

Types :
1. Descending inhibitory reticular projection.
2. Descending facilitatory reticular projection.

Functions :
1. Regulation of B.P., heart rate
2. Respiration control
3. Stretch reflexes
4. Amygdaloid nuceli
5. Stria terminalis

LIMBIC SYSTEM

Limbic system consist of :
1. Cingulate gyrus
2. Isthmus
3. Uncus
4. Hippocampal gyrus
5. Related subcortical nuclei
6. Amygdaloid nuclei
7. Stria terminalis

Functions

Limbic system controls :
1. Hunger and sex aspect
2. Memory
3. Heart rate, blood pressure
4. Motivation

BASAL GANGLIA

These are deep nuclie of the cerebral hemispheres.

These consists of :
1. Caudate nucleus
2. Putamen
3. Globus pallidus
4. Claustrum

Functionally subthalamic nuclie and the substantia nigra of midbrain and red nucleus are associated with the basal ganglia.

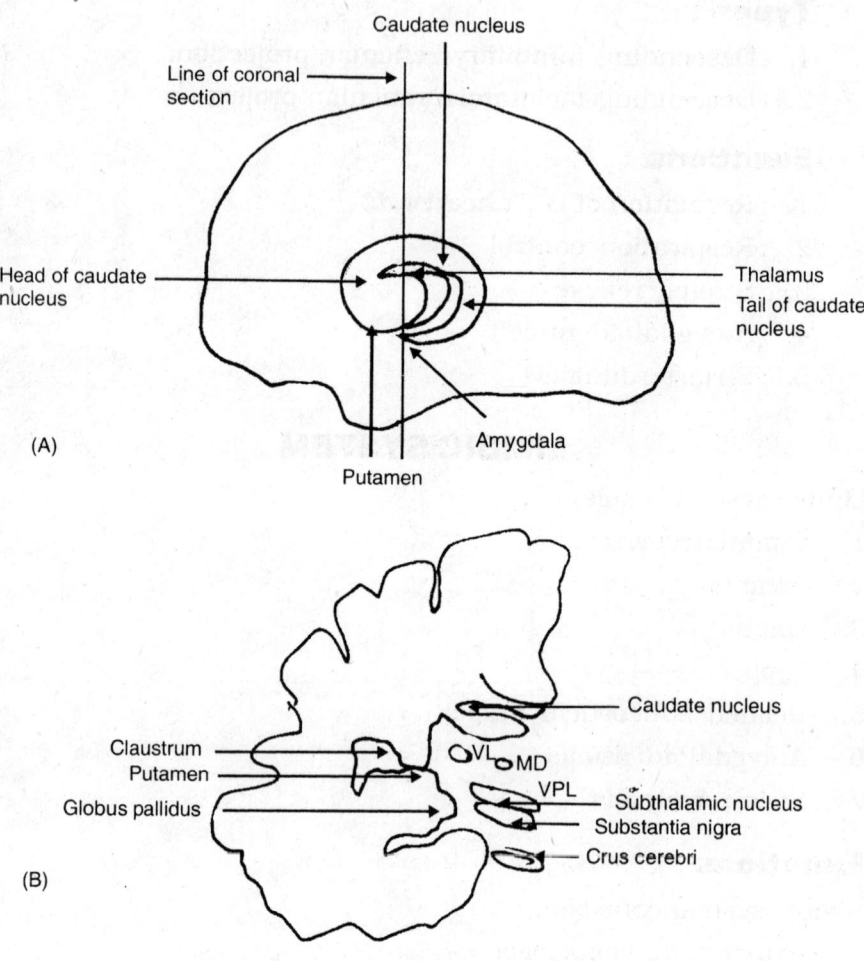

Fig. 13.13 The basal ganglia.

Connections of basal ganglia

This forms a loop. All parts of the cerebral cortex project to basal ganglia (corpus striatum). From putamen and caudate nuclei to globus pallidus, then to thalamus and back to cerebral cortex. The principal neural connections are depicted in the following diagram.

Functions of basal ganglia

1. Involved in basic patterns of movement. It plans the movements, represents motor programs formed in response to clues from cortex.

2. Subconscious gross movements.
3. Inhibition of stretch reflex.
4. Damage to basal ganglia leads to movement disorders. Parkinson's disease can occur.
5. Huntigton's chorea occurs due to basal ganglia disorders.

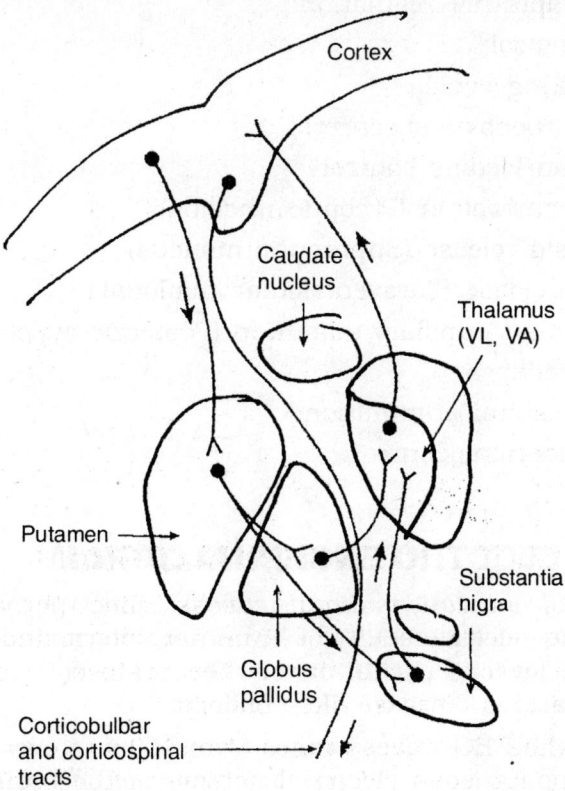

Fig. 13.14 Connections of basal ganglia.

HYPOTHALAMUS

Hypothalamus lies below the thalamus. It is composed of various nuclie.

Principle nuclie

1. Anterior nucleus
2. Preoptic nucleus
3. Paraventricular nucleus
4. Supraoptic nucleus
5. Arcuate nucleus

6. Ventromedial and dorsomedial nucleus
7. Posterior nucleus
8. Lateral nucleus

Principle functions

1. Control of circadian rhythm
2. Body temperature regulation
3. Thirst control
4. Sleep-waking cycle
5. Emotional behaviour control
6. Sateity and feeding control
7. Bladder contraction (Preoptic nucleus)
8. Vasopressin release (Supraoptic nucleus)
9. Oxytocin release (Paraventricular nucleus)
10. Shivering and pupillary dilatation (Posterior hypothalamus)
11. Feeding reflexes
12. Gastrointestinal stimulation
13. Neuroendocrinal control
14. Rage

ELECTRO ENCEPHALOGRAM

It is a record of undulations (brain waves). Since the pattern and intensity of the electric activity of brain are determined to a great extent by the level of excitation of the brain so it can help in detection of various diseases like epilepsy.

Amplitude of the EEG waves ranges from 10 μv to over 100 μv. It reflects the spontaneous electrical activity of the brain. Various factors affecting the appearance of EEG :

1. Age of the subject
2. The position of the electrodes
3. Behavioural state of the subject
4. Any organic disease

Much of the time the brain waves are irregular. Normal electro encephalogram consist of following waves.

Pattern

Alpha – Best seen over occipital lobe.
Beta – Normal awake pattern.
Theta – If seen in awake adults it is evidence of organic disease.

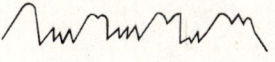 **Delta** – Deep sleep wave. If seen in the awake adults it is evidence of organic disease.

Methods of recording
1. Unipolar method
2. Bipolar method

Uses of EEG
1. Detection of organic diseases of brain like epilepsy.
2. Localization of subdural hematoma.

SLEEP

It is a physiological process by which bodily functions are rested.

The appearance of EEG can be used to follow the main stages of sleep. On starting of sleep theta waves occur, there may be periods of fast EEG activity with short periods of fast rhythmic waves known as sleep spindles. Deep sleep is dominated by large amplitude, low frequency, delta waves.

Sleep wakefullness cycle is an example of a 24 hour or circadian rhythm. Initiation of sleep occurs in the diencephalon and brainstem.

Types of sleep
1. Non-rapid eye movement sleep.
2. Rapid eye movement sleep.

Pattern of sleep changes with age. REM sleep decreases with age.

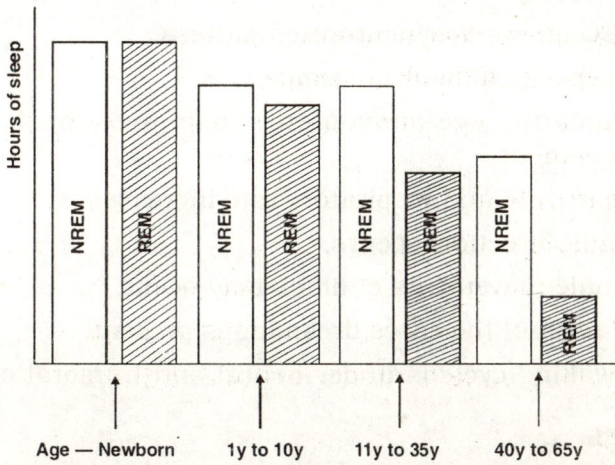

Fig. 13.15 With increasing age there is decrease in the hours of sleep and also the portion of REM sleep decreases with age.

Sleep cycle

Person willing to sleep
↓
Relaxed wakefullness
↓
Relaxed drowsiness
↓
Non-rapid eye movement sleep
↓
Rapid eye movement sleep
↓
Waking.

NREM sleep :
1. It consists of four stages :
   (a) Stage 1
   (b) Stage 2
   (c) Stage 3
   (d) Stage 4
2. Heart rate, respiratory rate decreases.
3. EEG pattern is of slower frequency and higher voltage.
4. Sleep spindles are characteristic.
5. Extensive relaxation of somatic muscle.

REM sleep :
1. EEG shows desynchronized pattern.
2. Sleeper is difficult to arouse.
3. Saccadic eye movements are present (rapid eye movement).
4. Heart rate and respiratory rate increases.
5. Penile erection occurs.
6. Clonic movements of limbs may occur.
7. In most of the cases dreaming is present.

Sleep waking cycle is under neural and humoral control.

Disorders

Insomnia : A condition in which a person is not able to sleep.

Sleep walking : Such individuals walk in sleep with their eyes open.

CEREBELLUM

It lies dorsal to the brain stem.

Parts of cerebellum

1. Vestibullo cerebellum
2. Spino cerebellum
3. Neo cerebellum

Cerebellum has about 30 million of functional units. This functional unit centres on a single very large purkinge cell. Cerebellar cortex consist of three major layers.

1. The molecular layer
2. Purkinge cell layer
3. Granule cell layer

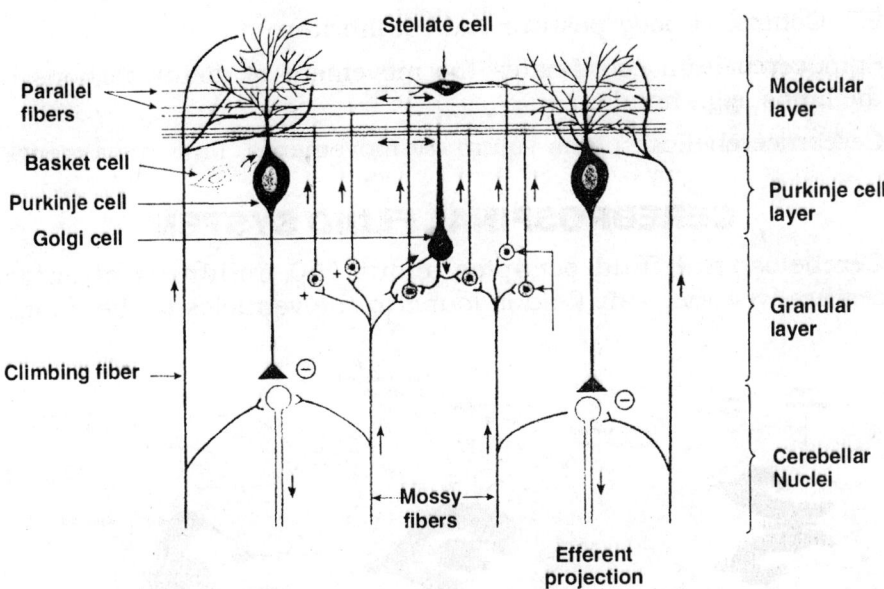

Fig. 13.16 The fundamental neural organization of the cerebellar cortex.

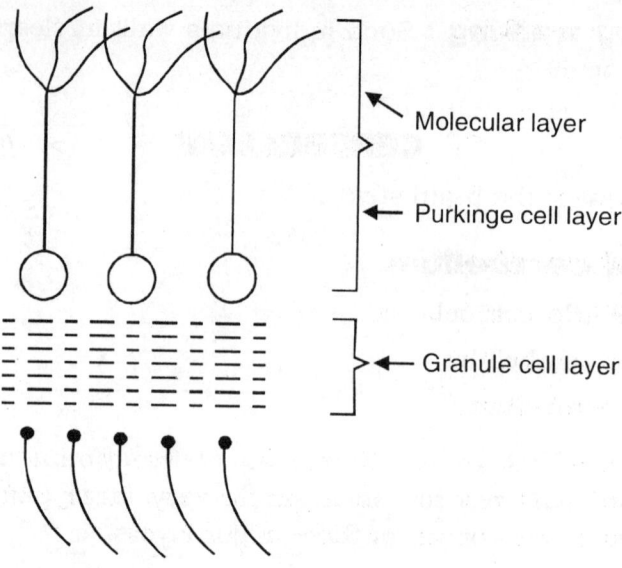

Fig. 13.17 Layers of cerebellar cortex.

Functions of the cerebellum

1. Control of movements
2. Control of body posture and equilibrium

Spinocerebellum coordinates the movement of distal portions of the limbs, e.g., hands.

Cerebrocerebellum plans voluntary movements, limb movements.

CEREBROSPINAL FLUID SYSTEM

Cerebelospinal fluid occupies about 150 milliliters of entire cerebral volume. This fluid is found in the venticles of the brain.

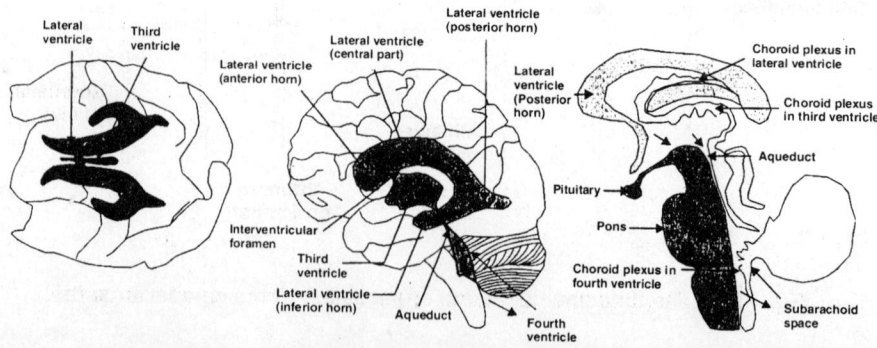

Fig. 13.18 Cerebrospinal fluid pathway. The black arrows show the pathway of cerebrospinal fluid flow from choroid in the lateral ventricles to the arachnoid villi.

Functions

Cushioning effect : It is the major function of the C.S.F. Brain floats in the cerebrospinal fluid. So that a blow to head moves the brain within the skull, preventing it from injury (Buffer effect).

Stable Ionic environment : C.S.F. is in direct contact with the extracellular fluid of the brain.

Composition of cerebrospinal fluid

Na^+ mmol^{-1}	141
K^+ mmol^{-1}	3
Ca^{2+} mmol^{-1}	1.2
Mg^{2+} mmol^{-1}	1.00
HCO_3^- mmol^{-1}	24
Protein (gl^{-1})	0.2
pH	8

Formation and circulation

About 500 ml of C.S.F. is formed each day by the choroid plexus in the lateral ventricles. The choroid plexus is a network of capillaries. C.S.F. flows from lateral ventricles to third ventricle than to aquiduct of silvius to IV ventricles. It comes out the IV ventricle via foramen of magendie and luschka and flows into subarachnoid space. Arachroid villi absorbs the C.S.F.

CONDITIONED REFLEXES

It is the ability to alter the behaviour on the basis of experience.

Characteristic features

The aquired reflexes or conditioned reflex are those reflex response to a stimulus that did not previously produce the responses; however, it developed by repeatedly pairing the stimulus with another stimulus that generally produce the response.

The classical example is Pavlov's classical dog experiment — Introduction of stimulus like ringing of bell produces no salivation in dog. But introduction of food into mouth sets up salivation. If ringing of bell was associated just before introduction of food, the ringing of bell produced salivation.

CIRCADIAN RHYTHM

The regular periodic nature of sleep-wakefulness cycle is an example of 24 hours or circadian rhythm. (Circa means *about* and dies means *day*).

Pineal gland is implecated to be responsible for circadian rhythm according to recent studies.

SPEECH

It is a means of communicating with fellow beings. Humans use language.

LEARNING

It is laying down of a store of knowledge. Memory is the name given to that store.

SOME IMPORTANT TERMS

1. Demyelination — Loss or destruction of myelin sheath around the neurons in the nervous system.
2. Neuropathy — Any disorder that affects the nervous system but particularly a disorder of cranial or spinal nerves.
3. Gullian Barre Syudrome — It is an acute demyelinating disorder in which axons of the peripheral nerves lose their myelin sheath.
4. Meningitis — Inflammation of meninges.
5. Neuralgia — Attack of pain along the course of a branch of a sensory nerve.
6. Neuritis — Inflammation of nerve.
7. Paresthesia — Abnormal sensation such as burning, pricking, tickling, tingling due to some disorder of sensory nerve.
8. Agnosia — Inabily to recognise the significance of sensory stimuls such as sounds, sight, smell, touch.
9. Encephalitis — An acute inflammation of brain.
10. Aprexia — Inability to carry out purposeful movements in the absence of paralysis.
11. Dementia — Progressive and permanent loss of intellectual abilities such as memory, judgement, abstract thinking.

14

THE SENSE ORGANS

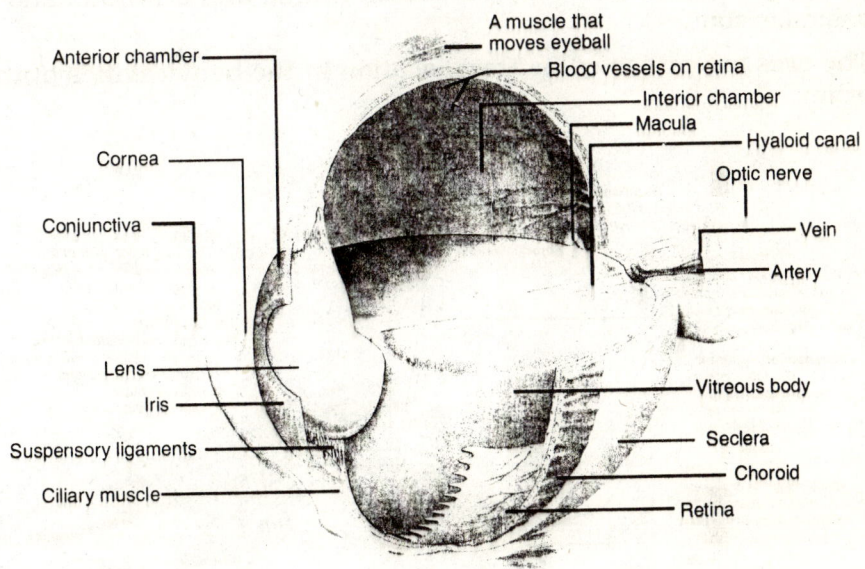

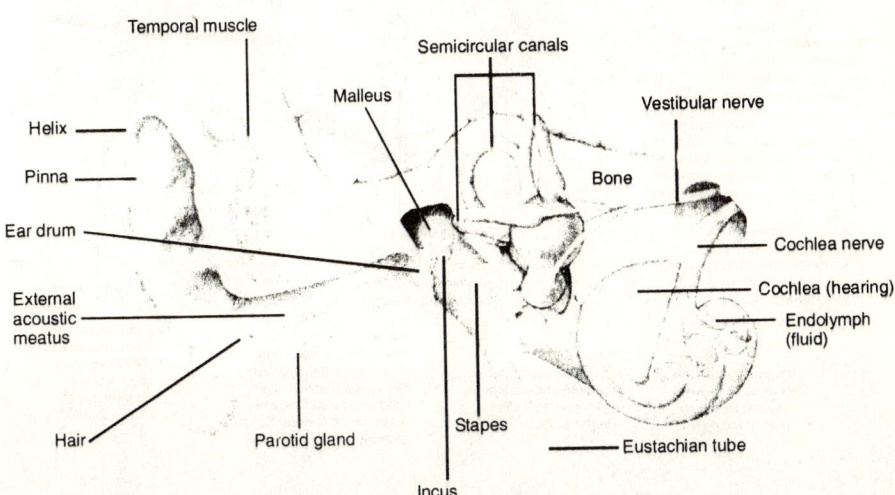

Fig. 14.1 Eye and ears.

THE EYE

Each eyeball is a cystic structure which is kept distended by the inside pressure. It has an anterior and a posterior pole.

Anteroposterior diameter : 24 mm

Horizontal diameter : 24 mm

Vertical diameter : 22 mm

Volume : 6.5 ml

Weight : 7 gm

The eyeball has a nervous coat called retina, and a fibrous and a vascular coat.

The eyes are protected by their location in the bony cavities of the orbits.

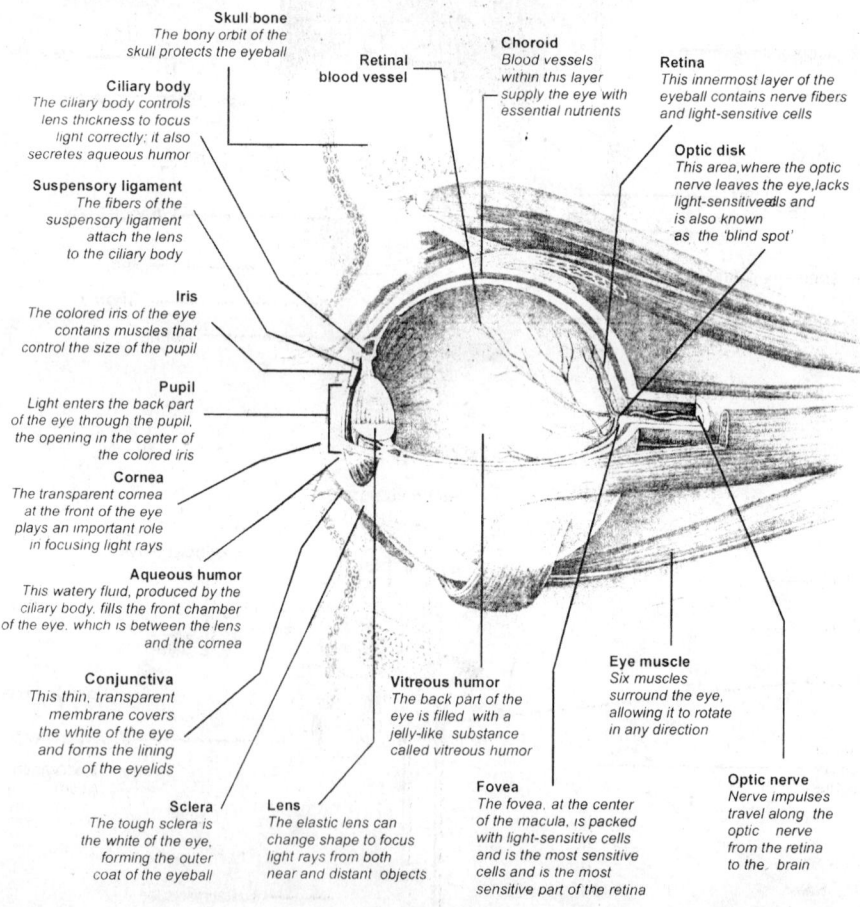

Fig. 14.2 Structure of eye.

The eyeball is roughly spherical and its wall consist of three layers:

Sclera — a tough outer coat

Choroid — a pigmented layer

Retina — a photoreceptor zone with nerve cells

Sclera appears white, choroid is under the sclera and it is highly vascular whereas retina contains photo-receptors.

Development of eye

The eyeball and its related structures are derived from neural ectoderm, mesoderm and ectoderm.

Ectoderm :
1. Lens
2. Corneal epithelium
3. Conjunctival epithelium
4. Lacrimal apparatus

Neural ectoderm :
1. Retina
2. Ciliary body
3. Pupillary muscle
4. Optic nerve

Mesoderm :
1. Walls of orbit
2. Blood vessels of choroid, iris, central retinal artery
3. The sclera

The lens

The lens is a transparent, biconvex, crystalline structure placed between iris and the vitreous. It has a diameter of 9-10 mm and thickness varies with age from 3.5 mm (at birth) to 5 mm (at extreme of age).

It contains lens capsule, anterior epithelium, lens fibres (nucleus and cortex), suspensory ligament.

The lens is a avascular structure and its metabolic activity is confined to the cortex and the nucleus is inert.

> **Cataract :** It is the disturbance in the transparency of the lens due to degenerative process, leading to lens opacification. Cataract may be congenital or acquired.

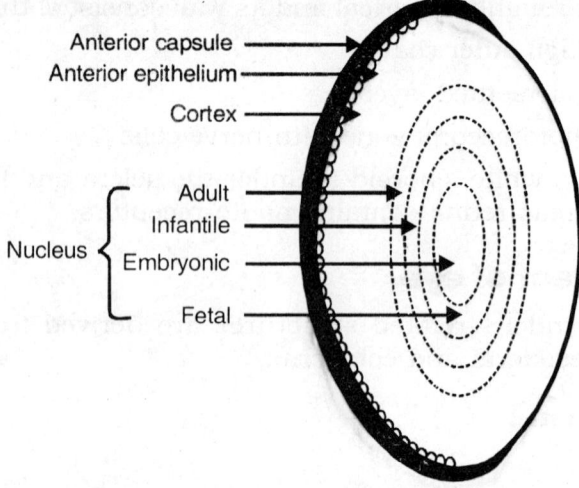

Fig. 14.3 Structure of lens.

The retina

It is the innermost layer of the eyeball.

Gross Anatomy : Retina extends from the optic disc to the ora serrate. It is divided into optic disc, macula and ora serrata as shown in the following diagram.

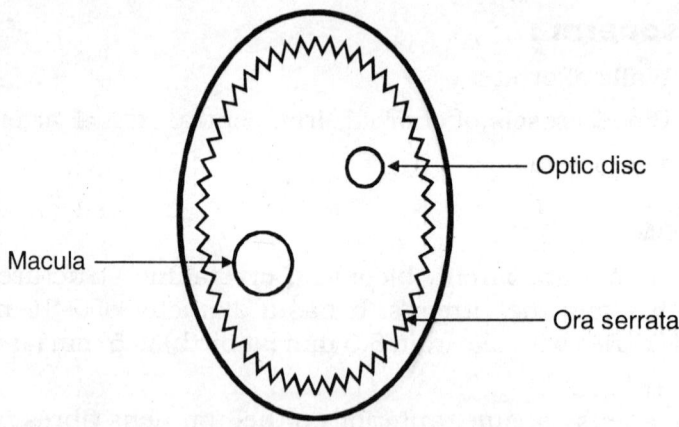

Fig. 14.4 Gross anatomy of the retina.

Microscopic structure : Retina has three type of cells and their synapses are arranged as following :

1. Pigment epithelium — outermost layer.

2. Rods and cones layer.
3. External limiting membrane.
4. Outer nuclear layer.
5. Outer plexiform layer.
6. Inner nuclear layer.
7. Inner plexiform layer.
8. Ganglion cell layer.
9. Nerve fibre layer.
10. Inner limiting layer.

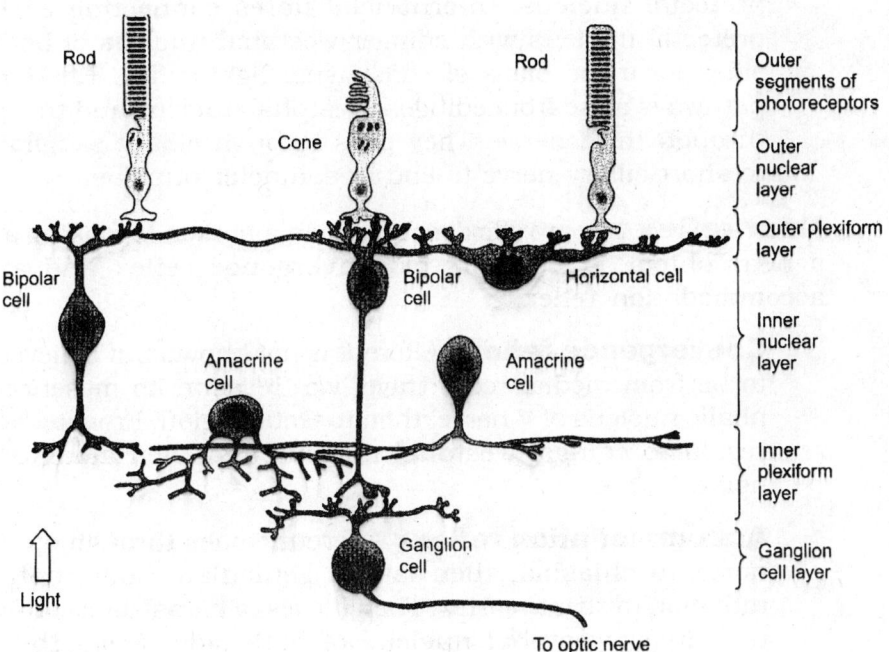

Fig. 14.5 Microscopic structure of retina.

The space between the cornea and the lens is filled with a clear fluid called aqueous humor, which supplies the lens and the cornea with nutrients.

The pressure within the eyeball is about 15 mmHg. It is known as intraocular pressure. It maintains eye rigidity. Light enters the eye via a clear zone known as cornea and it is focussed to retina by the lens.

The amount of light falling on the retina is controlled by the pupil.

Pulillary reflex

Light reflex : When light is thrown in one eye, both the pupils constrict. Constriction of pupil to which light is thrown is called direct light reflex and that of the other pupil is called consensual light reflex.

Pathways of light reflex : The afferent fibres extend from the retina to pretectal nucleus in the mid-brain. This passes along optic nerve to optic chiasma. Optic chiasma is the point where fibres from the nasal retina decussate and travel along the opposite optic tract to terminate in the contralateral pretectal nucleus. The temporal fibres are uncrossed and travel the same side to terminate on pretectal nucleus. Internuncial fibres connecting each pretectal nucleus with edinger-westphal nucleus of both sides form the basis of consensual light reflex. Efferent pathways arise from edinger- westphal nucleus and travel through third nerve. They pass through ciliary ganglion to short ciliary nerve to end in sphincter pupillae.

Near reflex : Near reflex occurs when a person is looking at a near object. It consists of convergence reflex and an accommodation reflex.

Convergence reflex : Afferent is not known but believed to be from medial recti, travel via 3rd nerve to mesencephalic nucleus of V nerve, then to tectal region. From tectal region to edinger-westphal nucleus and then along 3rd nerve.

Accommodation reflex : Afferent comes through optic nerve to chiasma, then lateral geniculate body, optic radiation to striate cortex. Then it goes to parastriate cortex to edinger-westphal nucleus of both side. From their travels along 3rd nerve to reach ciliary muscle and sphincter pupillae.

Blink reflex : It is reflex closure of eyelids from corneal irritation due to dust particles and other irritating substances.

Dazzle reflex : Very bright light causes closure of eyelids known as dazzle reflex.

Eye optics

Emmetropia : A state of refraction, when the parallel rays of light coming from infinity are focused at the sensitive layer of retina, when accommodation is at rest.

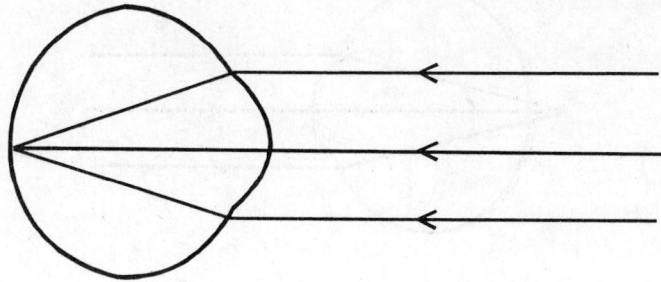

Fig. 14.6 Emmetropic eye.

Ametropia : A state of refraction, when the parallel rays of light coming from infinity (when accommodation is at rest) are focused either in front or behind the sensitive layer of retina in one or both the meridians.

It includes :
1. Hypermetropia
2. Myopia
3. Astigmatism

Hypermetropia : It is also known as long-sightedness. In this condition parallel rays of light coming from the infinity are focussed behind the retina when the accommodation is at rest.

Etiology :
1. *Axial hypermetropia* – axial shortening of eyeball.
2. *Curvatural hypermetropia* – curvature of cornea, lens or both is flatter.
3. *Index hypermetropia* – change is increase in the refractive index of the eye.
4. *Positional hypermetropia* – posterior placement of crystalline lens.

Symptoms : It may be asymptomatic or show asthenopic symptoms or defective vision only.

Complications :
1. Styes (recurrent)
2. Amblyopia
3. Accommodative convergent squint

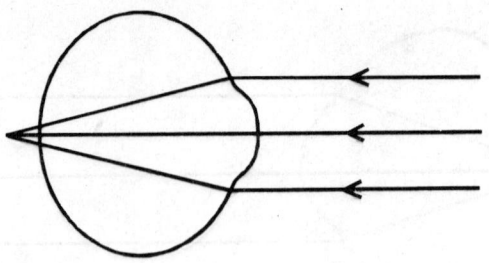

Fig. 14.7 Hypermetropic eye.

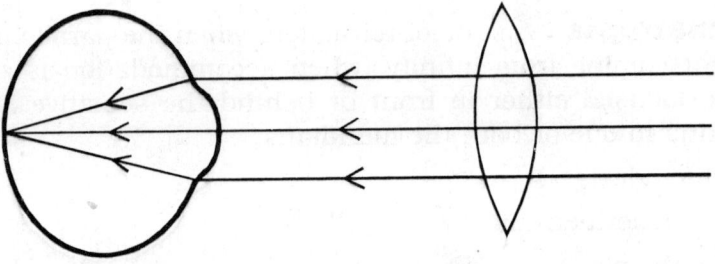

Fig. 14.8 Correction of hypermetropic eye using a conves lens.

Myopia : It is a type of refractive error in which parallel rays of light coming from the infinity are focused in front of the retina when accommodation is at rest.

Etiology :

1. *Axial myopia* — due to increase in anteroposterior length of the eyeball.
2. *Curvatural myopia* — due to increase in curuature of cornea, lens or both.
3. *Positional myopia* — due to anterior placement of crystalline lens in the eye.

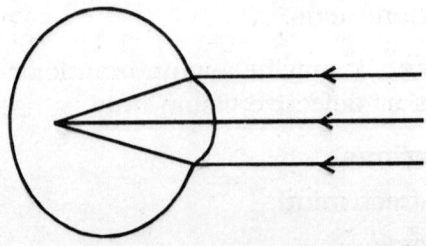

Fig. 14.9 Refraction of myopic eye.

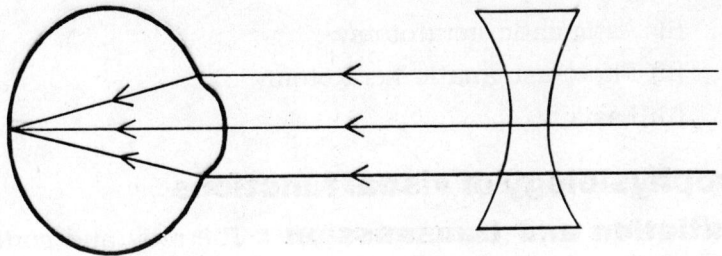

Fig. 14.10 Correction of myopic eye using a concave lens.

Symptoms : It shows defective vision, floating black spot may be seen. Night blindness and asthenopic symptoms can occur.

Treatment modalities for Hypermetropia and Myopia :

Hypermetropia :
1. Optical treatment — Convex lens.
2. Surgical treatment :
    (a) Hyperopic laser
    (b) Hyperopic lasik

Myopia :
1. Optical treatment – concave lens
2. Surgical treatment
    (a) Radial keratotomy
    (b) Photo refractive keratotomy
    (c) Lasik
    (d) Inter corneal ring implantation.

Astigmatism : In this type of refractive error the refraction varies in the different meridia.

Etiology :
1. *Corneal astigmatism* — due to curvature of cornea.
2. *Lenticular astigmatism* — lens induced due to curvature, refractive index.

Symptoms : Symptoms are from defective vision, object blurring, to asthenopic symptoms.

Treatment :
Optical treatment — cylindrical lens are prescribed.

Surgical treatment:

(i) Astigmatic keratotomy

(ii) Photo-astigmatic keratotomy

(iii) Lasik

Neurophysiology of visual functions

Initiation and transmission : The rods and cones are the sensory nerve endings for visual sensation. Light falling upon the retina causes photo-chemical and electrical reaction. These electrical reactions pass through nerve fibres to the brain.

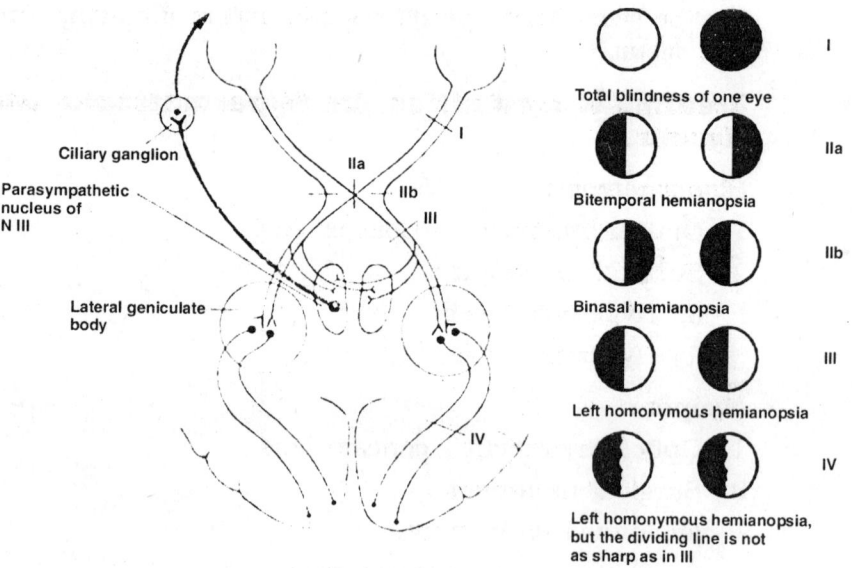

Fig. 14.11 The visual pathways. Damage to the tracts at the locations indicated causes defects in the visual fields as shown in the diagrams on the right.

Perception : It is an integration of light sense, form sense, contrast sense and colour sense.

Light sense : Sense of awareness of light is known as light sense.

Dark adaptation : It is the ability of eye to abopt itself to decreasing illumination.

Dark adaptation time : When one goes from a bright light to a dark room, he cannot see the objects at that time, but is able to make out after some time. This time interval is known as dark adaptation time. Initial dark adaptation is due to cones and rest is rods.

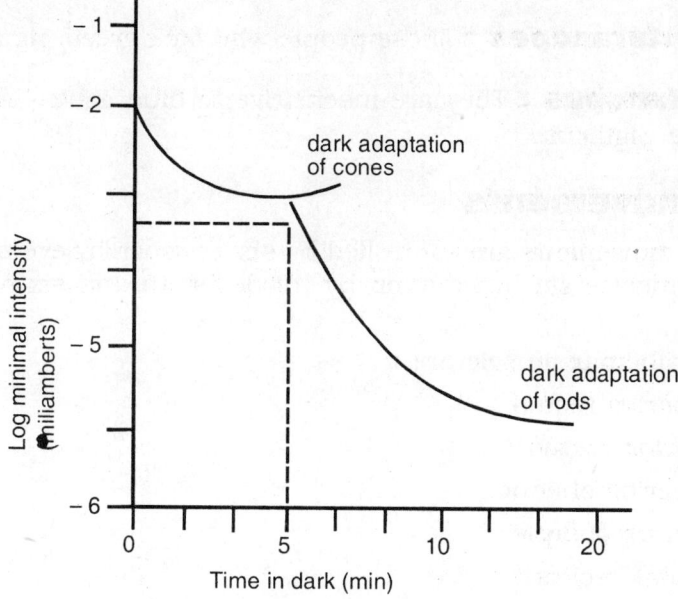

Fig. 14.12 Dark adaptation.

Photopic vision — Cones are sensitive to bright light, so they are used more in bright light. The vision due to cones is called photopic vision.

Scotopic vision — Rods are sensitive to dim light, so they are used more in dim light. The vision due to rods is called scotopic vision.

Form sense : It is the ability to discriminate between the shapes of the object. It is due to cones.

Contrast sense : It is the ability to perceive slight changes in the luminance.

Colour sense : It is the ability of the eye to differentiate between different colours. It is due to cones.

Colour blindness

There are three type of cones, each being sensitive to a particular wavelength. Some people have defective cone pigments and are said to be color blind.

The most common are the trichromats who match colours with unusual proportions of red and green. True color blind are those people who lack one or other cone pigment.

Protanopes : Those people who lack red pigment.

Deuteranopes : Those people who lack green pigment.

Tritanopes : They are insensitive to blue light – they lack blue pigment.

Eye movements

The eye movements are controlled by six extraocular eye muscles. These muscles get innervation by third, fourth and sixth cranial nerves.

The extraocular muscle are :

1. Superior rectus
2. Inferior rectus
3. Superior oblique
4. Inferior oblique
5. Medial rectus
6. Lateral rectus

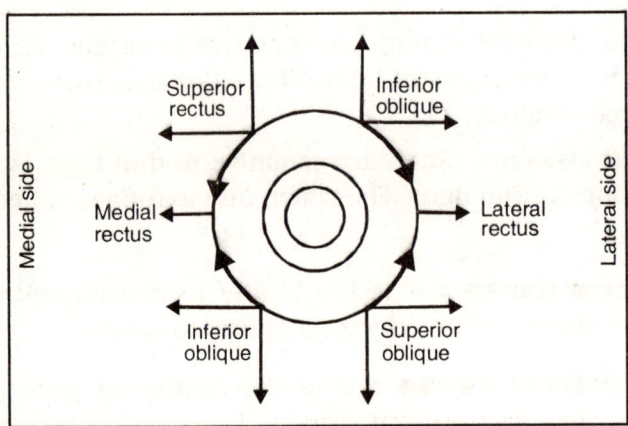

Fig. 14.13 Various extraocular muscles producing movements of the eyeball.

Accomodation

The light rays reflected from an object closer than 6 m diverge, leading to the blurring of the object. This is saved by increasing the refractive power of lens by a process called accommodation.

When at rest the circular lens ligament pulls the lens into a flattened shape, while looking at a near object the ciliary muscle contracts causing decrease in tension on lens which makes lens more convex. This is the basic principle of accommodation.

In a child with normal vision, the refractive power of eye can increase to upto ≈ 74 D by means of accommodation.

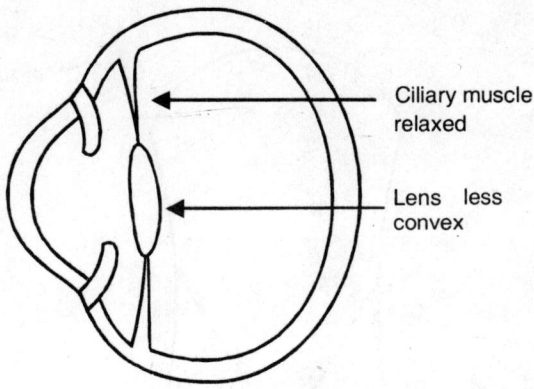

Fig. 14.14 Accommodation at rest.

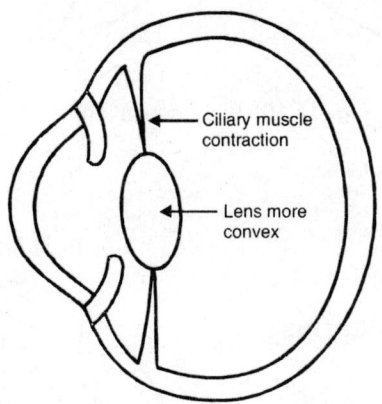

Fig. 14.15 Accommodation.

TASTE

The receptors for taste are present in taste buds which are located in the walls of papillae of the tongue and in the mucosa of the palate and pharynx.

There are four types of papillae in the mucous membrane of the tongue :

1. Fusiform papillae
2. Vallate papillae
3. Foliate papillae
4. Filiform papillae

The receptors are hair cells. These receptors are continuously replaced. The chemical substance dissolved in the saliva elicit impulses. Anterior 2/3 of tongue are transmitted by VII nerve. Post 1/3 of tongue is transmitted by IX nerve.

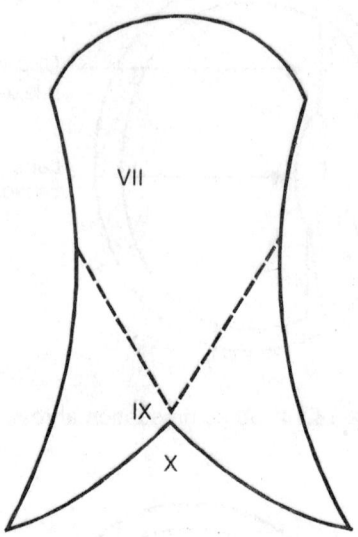

Fig. 14.16 Taste sensation.

Neural pathway

VII, IX, X nerve
↓
Nucleus of tractus solitarius
↓
Medial leminiscus
↓
Thalamus
↓
Brain stem

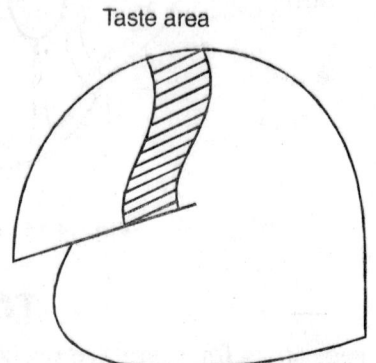

Fig. 14.17 Neural pathway.

Basic taste sensations

1. Tip of tongue is for sweet sensation.
2. Back of tongue is for bitter taste.
3. Side of tongue is for sour sensation.
4. Dorsum of tongue is for salt sensation.

General sensation (other than taste)

1. Anterior 2/3 of tongue : V nerve.
2. Posterior 1/3 of tongue : IX nerve.

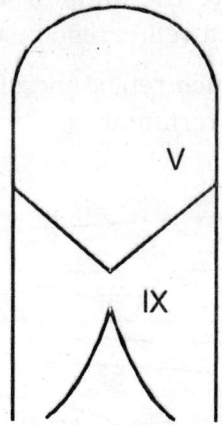

Fig. 14.18 General sensation (other than taste).

SMELL

The receptors for smell are located in the olfactory epithelium.

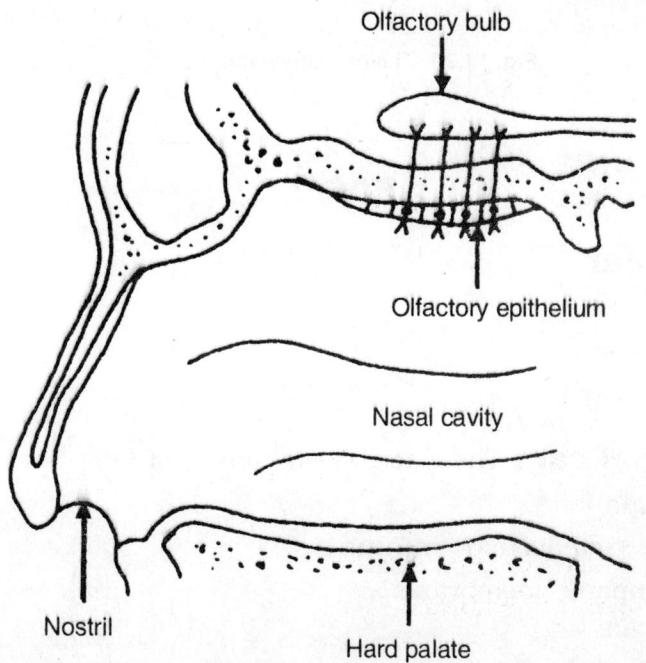

Fig. 14.19 Olfactory apparatus.

The olfactory receptor cells are bipolar neurons. Their axons pass through the perforation of cribriform plate of ethmoid bone. They enter olfactory bulb then to mitral cells and in turn olfactory tract.

Olfactory tract transmits olfactory impulses to the primary olfactory cortex. Odorous particle are the initiator of stimuli. They secrete saliva and gastric juice as a reflex response.

Irritating substances produce reflex sneezing and tears secretion via somatic sensory nerve terminal.

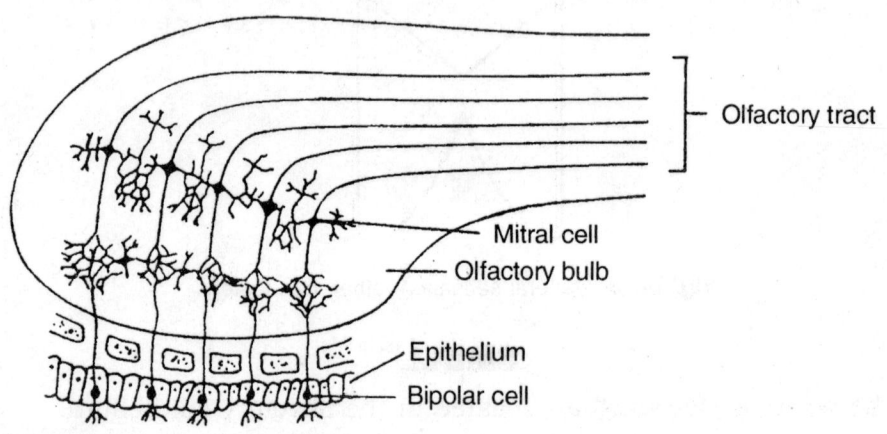

Fig. 14.20 The olfactory pathway.

EAR

Parts of ear
1. External ear
2. Middle ear
3. Internal ear

External ear : The external ear consist of :
(a) Pinna
(b) External acoustic meatus
(c) Tympanic membrane

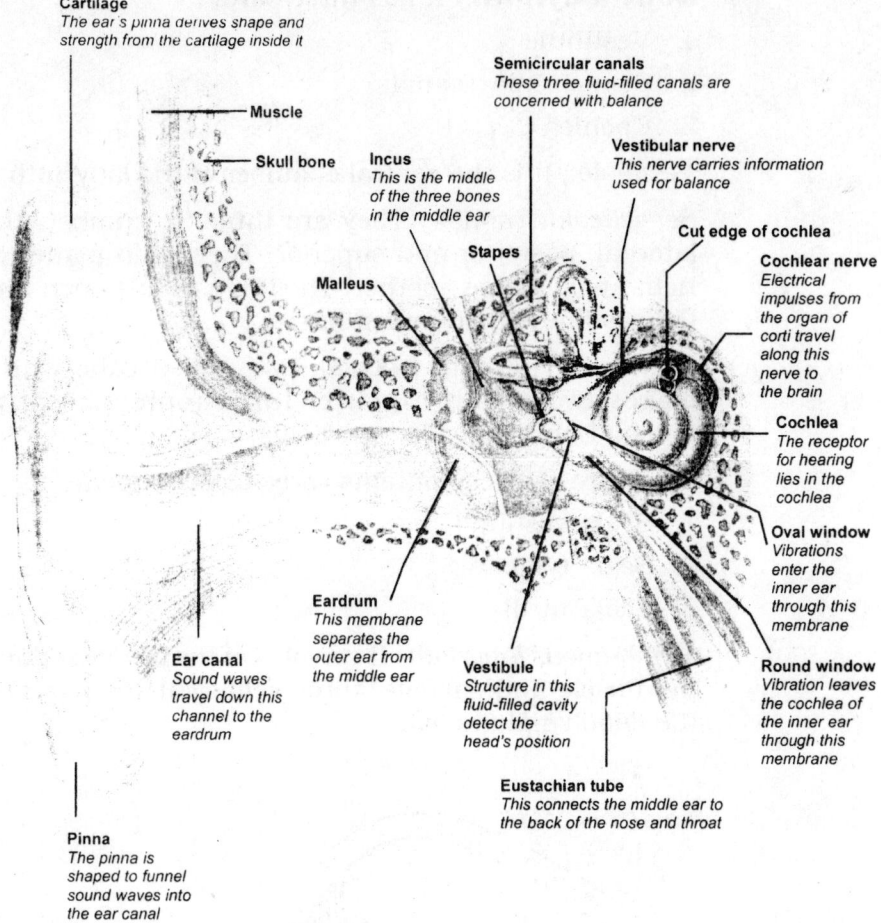

Fig. 14.21 Components of the ear.

Middle ear : Middle ear together with the eustachian tube, aditus, antrum and mastoid aircells is called the middle ear cleft.

There are three ossicles in the middle ear :

(a) The malleus
(b) The incus
(c) The stapes

Internal ear : The internal ear or the labyrinth is an organ of hearing and balance.

It has a bony and a membranous labyrinth. The mem-branous labyrinth is filled with endolymph while the space between membranous and bony labyrinth is filled with perilymph.

Bony labyrinth : It has three parts :
1. Vestibule
2. Semicircular canals
3. Cochlea

Vestibule : It is the central chamber of the labyrinth.

Semicircular canals : They are three in number; the laternal, posterior and superior. They lie in planes at right angle to one another. The three canals open into the vestibule by five openings.

Cochlea : The bony cochlea is a coiled tube which makes two to three quarter turns round a central pyramid of bone called modiolus.

The bony cochlea contains three compartments :
1. Scala vestibuli.
2. Scala tympani.
3. Scala media.

Membranous labyrinth : It consists of the cochlear duct, the utricle and saccule, three semicirular ducts and the endolymphatic sac.

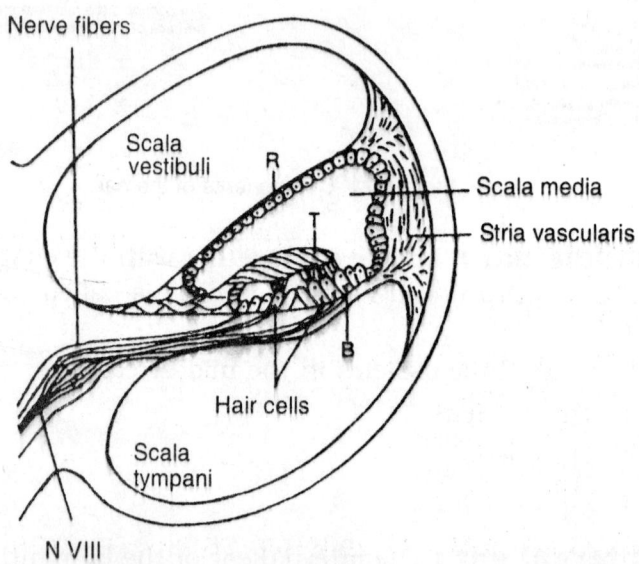

Fig. 14.22 Section through cochlea showing the three compartments.
R – Reissuer's membrane
B – Basilar membrane
T – Tectorial membrane

Auditory system

The auditory system may be divided into:

Central auditory system : It consist of the neural pathways concerned with the analysis of sound impulses from the cochlear nuclei to auditory system.

Peripheral auditory system : It consist of ear, the auditory nerve and the neurons of the spiral ganglia.

The outer and middle ear serves to collect sound energy and focus it to the oval window. This transfers sound energy to the cochlea.

Incident sound waves cause pressure waves to be set up in the fluid of the cochlea.

These pressure waves cause travelling wave in the basilar membrane that activates hair cells which is responsible for sound transduction.

Higher frequency are presented near to the apex of the cochlea. The number of action potential in a specific fiber codes for the intensity of the sound.

Applied Physiology

Conductive deafness : Hearing loss from a defect in the middle to outer ear.

Sensorineural hearing loss : When some part of cochlea or auditory nerve is damaged sensorineural hearing loss occurs.

THE LARYNX

Anatomy of larynx

It is an organ for production of voice. It's also an air passage and acts as a sphincter at the inlet of the lower respiratory passage.

It lies in the anterior midline of the neck, extending from the root of the tongue to the trachea.

It is made up of skeletal frame work of cartilages which are 9 in number of which 3 are paried and 3 are unpaired.

Unpaired cartilages :
1. Thyroid
2. Cricoid
3. Epiglottic

Paired cartilages :
1. Arytenoid
2. Corniculate
3. Cuneiform

During speech, the glottis is reduced to a chink by the adduction of the vocal folds.

During whispering, the intermembranous part of the rima glottidis is closed.

The formation of the language is controlled by wernicke's area which lies behind the primary auditory cortex in the posterior part of the superior gyrus of the temporal lobe.

Broca's area is the special area in the frontal cortex which provides the neural circuitary for word formation. It works in close association with wernicke's language centre.

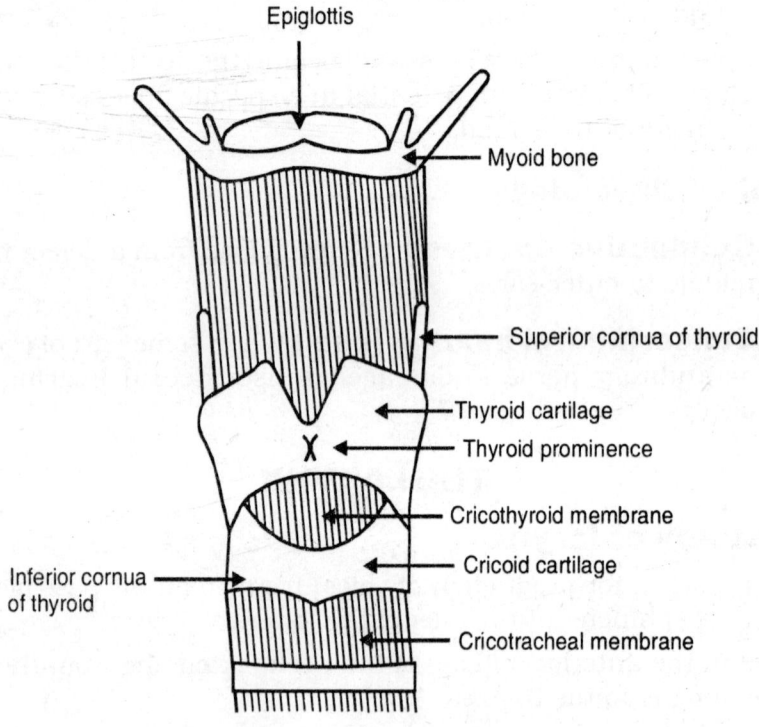

Fig. 14.24 The laryngeal framework.

Speech

It is a very complex skill. It requires very precise motor acts to produce specific sounds in correct order. The precise regulation of flow of air through the larynx and mouth is required.

Brain area controlling speech : Speech is localized to the left hemisphere in the majority of the population. In the temporal lobe there is a wernicke's area which originates speech.

The neural codes for production of speech pass via the arcuate fasciculus to Broca's area for appropriate motor action.

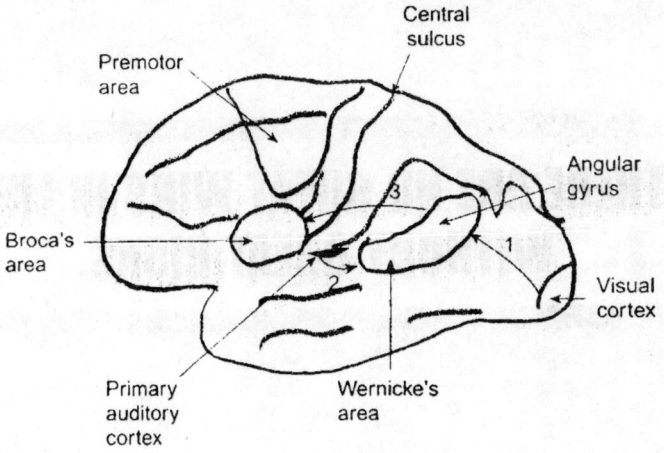

Fig. 24 A diagram of the left hemisphere to show the location of the principal regions involved in the control of speech. 1 & 2 indicate the postulated connections between the primary visiual and auditory receiving area, and the language areas of the temporal lobe and angular gyrus. 3 indicates the connection between the angular gyrus and broca's area via the arcuate fasciculus.

Applied physiology : Aphasia occurs due to damage to Broca's area or speech areas.

THERE ARE NO GREAT WINS IN LIFE WITHOUT GREAT RISKS.

15

ENDOCRINE SYSTEM

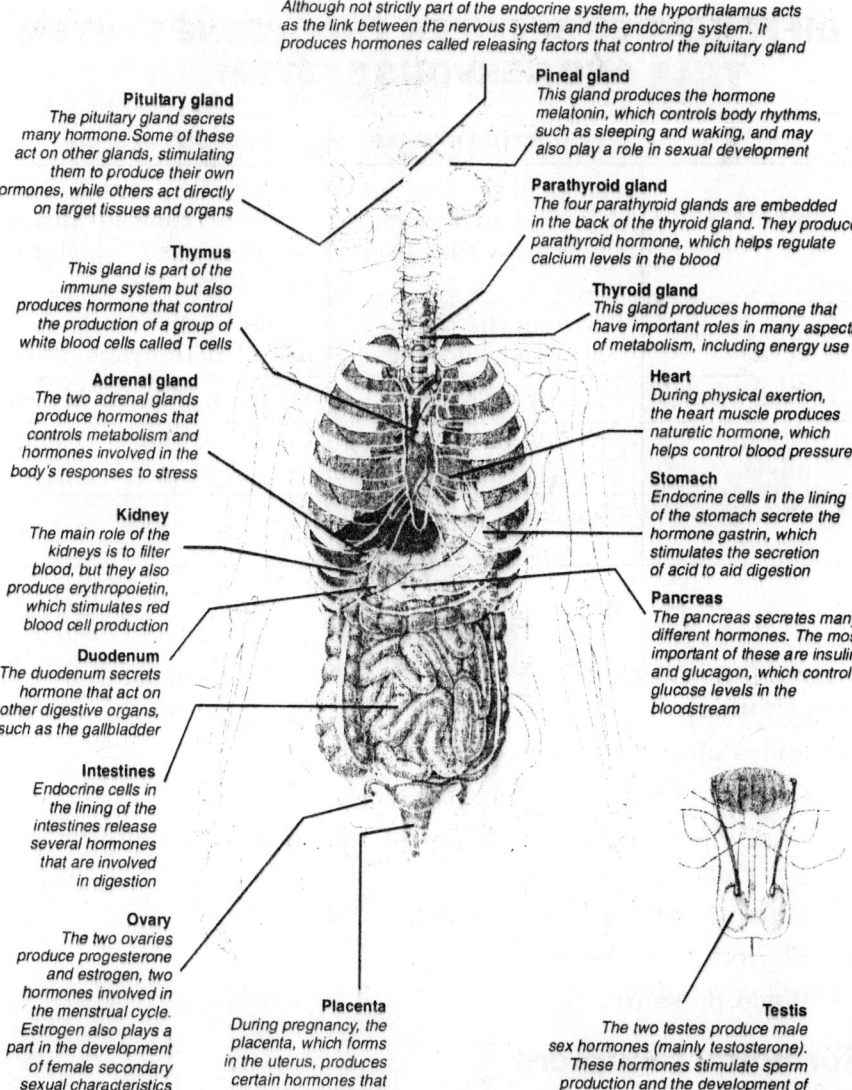

Hypothalamus
Although not strictly part of the endocrine system, the hypothalamus acts as the link between the nervous system and the endocrine system. It produces hormones called releasing factors that control the pituitary gland

Pituitary gland
The pituitary gland secrets many hormone. Some of these act on other glands, stimulating them to produce their own hormones, while others act directly on target tissues and organs

Pineal gland
This gland produces the hormone melatonin, which controls body rhythms, such as sleeping and waking, and may also play a role in sexual development

Thymus
This gland is part of the immune system but also produces hormone that control the production of a group of white blood cells called T cells

Parathyroid gland
The four parathyroid glands are embedded in the back of the thyroid gland. They produce parathyroid hormone, which helps regulate calcium levels in the blood

Thyroid gland
This gland produces hormone that have important roles in many aspects of metabolism, including energy use

Adrenal gland
The two adrenal glands produce hormones that controls metabolism and hormones involved in the body's responses to stress

Heart
During physical exertion, the heart muscle produces naturetic hormone, which helps control blood pressure

Kidney
The main role of the kidneys is to filter blood, but they also produce erythropoietin, which stimulates red blood cell production

Stomach
Endocrine cells in the lining of the stomach secrete the hormone gastrin, which stimulates the secretion of acid to aid digestion

Duodenum
The duodenum secrets hormone that act on other digestive organs, such as the gallbladder

Pancreas
The pancreas secretes many different hormones. The most important of these are insulin and glucagon, which control glucose levels in the bloodstream

Intestines
Endocrine cells in the lining of the intestines release several hormones that are involved in digestion

Ovary
The two ovaries produce progesterone and estrogen, two hormones involved in the menstrual cycle. Estrogen also plays a part in the development of female secondary sexual characteristics

Placenta
During pregnancy, the placenta, which forms in the uterus, produces certain hormones that are essential for fetal development

Testis
The two testes produce male sex hormones (mainly testosterone). These hormones stimulate sperm production and the development of male secondary sexual characteristics

Fig. 15.1 Hormone secreting glands and cells.

INTRODUCTION

Billions of cells of the human body communicate with one another to synchronise their activities. Adjacent cells communicate via molecules produced by them which effect the activities of neighbouring cells. Communication between cells over longer distance is via nervous or endocrine system.

Endocrine system consists of endocrine glands. These are called so as they release their secretions directly into blood. Also called ductless glands because they do not posses excretory ducts.

DIFFERENCES BETWEEN ENDOCRINE SYSTEM AND NERVOUS SYSTEM

	Endocrine system	Nervous system
1. How mediated	Mediated by hormones delivered to tissues in the body by the blood	Mediated by neurotransmitters released locally in response to nerve impulses.
2. Site of action	Far from the site of release of hormone	Close to the site of release of neurotransmitter.
3. Target cells	All body cells	Muscles, glands, nerves.
4. Duration of onset	Seconds to hours or days	Usually within a fraction of a second.
5. Duration of action	Longer	Brief.

HORMONES

Derived from Greek word hormaein which means – to set in motion or to stimulate.

Hormones play major roles in :
1. Cellular synthesis, secretion.
2. Anabolism and catabolism of carbohydrates, lipids and proteins.
3. Mineral and water metabolism.
4. Reproduction.
5. Blood pressure.

Hormonal receptors

These receptors are located on target cell membrane or located within the cytoplasm and nucleus of the target cell.

Generally a target cell contains 2000 to 1,00,000 receptors.

Classes of hormones

1. Protein and proteinaceous hormones
2. Steroid hormones

Proteinaceous hormones are sub classified into :

(a) Amino acid derivatives. E.g. adrenaline and noradrenaline (catecholamines).
(b) Iodinated amino acid derived hormones. E.g. Thyroxine.
(c) Peptide hormones — Contains two to ten amino acids. E.g. vasopressin, angiotensin II.
(d) Polypeptide hormones — Contains less than 100 amino acids. E.g. glucagon and insulin.
(e) Protein hormones — Contains 100 or more amino acids. E.g. GH and thyrotropin.

Classification of hormones by chemical class

		Hormone	Site of Secretion
1.	**Lipid Soluble**		
	(a) Steroid	Aldosterone Cortisal Androgens	Adernal contex.
		Testosterone	Testes.
		Estrogen Progesterone	Ovaries.
	(b) Thyroid Hormones	T_3 (triiodothyronine) T_4 (thyroxine)	Thyroid gland.
2.	**Water Soluble**		
	(a) Amines	Epinephrine and norepinephrine	Adrenal medulla.
		Melatonin	Pineal gland.
		Serotonin	Platelets.
		Histamine	Mast cells.
	(b) Peptides and Proteins	Hypothalamic releasing and inhibitory hormones	Hypothalamus.
		Oxytocin Antidiuretic hormone	Posterior pituitary.
		Growth hormone Thyroid stimulating hormone ACTH Follicle stimulating hormone Luteinising hormone Prolactin	Anterior pituitary.

	Insulin / Glucagon / Somatostatin	Pancreas.
	Parathyroid hormone	Parathroid glands.
	Calcitonin	Thyroid gland.
	Gastrin / Secretin / Cholecystokinin	Stomach and small intestine.
	GIP Erythropoietin	Kidneys.
(c) Eicosanoids	Prostaglandins / Leuko trienes	All body cells except red blood cells.

Prohormones / preprohormones : Some of the peptides and polypeptide hormones are split products of larger protein molecules. They are inactivated form of hormones.

Mechanism of hormone action

1. Hormone binds to its receptors on the cell membrane activating the receptor.
2. G proteins bind to activated receptors and is itself activated.
3. G protein activates by reacting with adenylate cyclase present on cell surface (inner).
4. Via cAMP dependent protein kinase enzyme.

HYPOTHALAMUS

It is organized in a number of nuclei out of which supraoptic nucleus mainly produces ADH.

Oxytocin is mainly produced by paraventricular nucleus. The medial eminence outside blood brain barrier is associated with the portal system.

It is connected with higher brain centres, e.g., cerebral cortex. Also with spinal cord and peripheral organs.

Neurohypophysis is connected with hypothalmus by hypothalamo hypophysial tract.

Adenohypophysis is connected via hypothalamo hypophysial portal system.

Functions

Neurogenic and endocrine.

Neurogenic :

1. Acts as a higher centre of autonomic nervous system.

2. It is a centre for exteriosation of emotion.
3. It is a centre for control of body temperature.
4. It is a centre for hunger and satiety sensations.
5. It is involved in control of blood pressure.
6. It controls adrenaline secretion.

Endocrine : It synthesises ADH, oxytocin, regulatory peptides etc.

ADH :
1. It is a non-peptide hormone produced in supraoptic nucleus. Its secretion is controlled by osmoreceptors, volume receptors, chemoreceptors and by higher centres.
2. Its actions are mainly :
    (a) Increased permeability of distal renal tubules to H_2O.
    (b) Increased reabsorption of H_2O from distal tubules.
    (c) Increased blood pressure.

Oxytocin :
1. It is a non-peptide produced by paraventricular nucleus. Secretion is controlled by *reflexes*, e.g., milk let down reflex, by touch receptors, e.g., in the areola.
2. Actions :
    1. Stimulates milk ejection.
    2. Stimulates uterus contraction.
    3. Also it is involved in parturition.

Regulatory peptides :
1. It includes thyroliberin, somatoliberin, corticoliberin, somatostatin etc.
2. Secretion is controlled by higher brain centres and by tropic hormones of pituitary.
3. Functions :
    (a) Control releases of tropic hormones.
    (b) Deficiency or excess causes pathophysiology.

PITUITARY GLAND

1. Anterior pituitary
2. Posterior pituitary

Posterior pituitary (neurohypophysis)

It stores and releases ADH and oxytocin and produces enkephalins and it is connected to hypothalamus by hypothalamo hypophysial tract.

Anterior pituitary (adenohypophysis)

It is divided into anterior, middle and tuberal lobes (dominant).

Anterior lobe has chromophils :

1. Acidophils – 35% secrete GH (growth hormone) and Prolactin.
2. Basophils – 15% secrete TT, CT, FT, MT and BLPH.

Chromophobes : 50% of cells stans pale.

GH or somatotropin :

1. Promotes trans membrane transport of amino acids.
2. Stimulates protein synthesis and cellular growth.
3. Stimulates linear growth in long bones.
4. Stimulates thickening of bones.
5. Anti-insulin effect.
6. Causes Ca^{2+}, Pi and Na^+ retention.
7. Excess causes gigantism or acromegaly. Deficiency in children causes pituitary dwarfism.

Prolactin :

1. Stimulates lactogenesis.
2. Suppresses gonadotropin secretion.
   (Dopamine) inhibits secretion.
3. Excess causes lactorrhea in both sexes.

Thyrotropin (TSH) :

1. Determines size of the thyroid.
2. Controls every phase of thyroid function.
3. Over production causes hyperthyroidism
4. Under production causes :
   (a) Cretinism in young
   (b) Myxoedema in adults

Melanotropin (MSH) :
Controls skin colour in reptiles, fishes. In humans function unclear.

ACTH :
1. Regulates secretion of adrenocortical hormones
2. Excess causes cushing's syndrome
3. Deficiency causes addison's diseases
4. Control by negative feedback.

Gonadotropins (FSH & LH) :
1. FSH stimulates ovogenesis and spermatogenesis.
2. LH stimulates female and male hormone secretion.
3. Control by circulating sex hormones by feedback on anterior lobe.
4. Any endocrinopathy causes menstrual disturbances and sterility.

THYROID GLAND

It produces two types of hormones :
1. Iodothyronines
2. Calcitonin

Iodothyronines or thyroid hormones are mainly T_4 and T_3. Their functions are as follows :
1. Stimulates metabolism of most cells.
2. Increase demand for O_2 and raise Basal Metabolic Rate.
3. Promotes glucose absorption and catabolism.
4. Stimulates lipolysis or catabolism of lipids.
5. Derangement of thyroid function causes simple goiter or endemic goitre.

Hypothyroidism
1. Two types cretinism and myxoedema.
2. Both types characterised by low BMR, cold intolerance, a dry thick skin, bradycardia, hyperlipidemia etc.
3. Cretinism is associated with dwarfism and mental retardation.

Hyperthyroidism
1. Caused by thyroid stimulating immunoglobulins.
2. Characterised by diffuse enlargement of thyroid, tachycardia, warm skin, sweating, nervousness, irritability, weight loss, exophthalmos etc.

3. Secondary type caused by hyperfunctioning nodules. Hyperactivity independent of excess thyrotropin or TSIS.

Parathormone, Calcitonin, Vitamin-D

The total body calcium is approximately 1,100 gm (27.5 mol). Its distribution is 99% in skeleton and only 1% in extra-skeletal (1%). In skeleton 98% is present as hydroxyapatite crystals and 2% as $CaHPO_4$. Extraskeletal to intraskeletal ratio is more than 1000:1. In plasma, 2.5 mmol/l and 50% ionised form is present.

The daily intake is 18.75 mmol and various sources are dairy products, which is an excellent source. The other sources are Vitamin-D which is abrobed in proximal small intestine and parathormone promotes this absorption.

Lack of bile salts and lipase decreases this absorption.

Homeostasis is regulated by parathormone, calcitonin and Vitamin-D. And it has inverse relationship between plasma Calcium and Phosphate levels.

Parathyroids : Ca^{2+} is required for calcification, enzyme activation, hormone and transmitter release etc.

Hypercalcaemia : Parathormone or Vitamin-D excess, bone metastasis, etc.

Source of parathormone is parathyroid glands located on posterior aspect of thyroid and are four in number. Its secretion is controlled by plasma $[Ca^{2+}]$, its decrease stimulates secretion. Its biosynthesis consists of 3 steps : Preparathormone – Proparathormone – Parathormone. Its action consists of stimulation of intestinal absorption of Ca^{2+} indirectly, stimulates reabsorption of Ca^{2+} in distal renal tubules, promotes urinary exeration of phosphates. It also activates 1 α hydroxylase and thus calcitriol production. Its high concentration stimulates bone resorption by osteoclasts.

Hyper parathyroidism is characterised by respotion of bone, hypercalcaemia and hypophosphatemia, kidney stones and calcifications, spontaneous fractures, pain, etc.

Hypoparathyroidism is characterised by hypocalcaemia, hyperphosphataemia and tetany. It is caused by hypoparathyroidism or Vitamin-D deficiency.

Vitamin D-3 (Cholecalciferol) : Its source is food and is also synthesized in skin from 7 – dehydrocholesterol.

Vitamin-D and its derivatives are steroids. It is hydroxylated at

C-25 in the liver (Calcidiol) with t½ = 15 hours. 25 OH - D_3 is hydroxylated at C_1 in kidney to 125 $(OH)_2 D_3$ (calcitriol) with $t_{½}$ = 15 d. Enzyme 1α – hydoxylase is activated by parathormone. It stimulates Ca^{2+} and phosphate absoption from intesetine, promotes reabsorption of Ca^{2+} and phosphate from renal tubules. Normal concentration of the vitamin promotes calcification; high doses of the vitamin stimulates bone resorption. Its deficiency causes avitaminosis D producing rickets in children, osteomalacia in adults, plasma calcium and phosphate levels are decreased, newly formed tissue fails to calcify, also causes skeletal malformation, pain, muscle weakness. If it is present in excess caused by therapeutic and biosynthetic excess is known as hyper vitaminosis D characterised by hypercalemia, hyper-phosphataemia, anorexia, calcification of soft tissues etc.

Bone physiology : It is a living, calcified osteoid tissue. Its main functions are :

1. They act as levers for muscles and support the body,
2. Protect vital organs : brain, heart, etc.
3. Involved in maintaining acid base balance
4. Help to maintain calcium homeostasis.

Bone formation occurs by intramembranous and endochondral mechanism and its growth is linear occurring at epiphysial cartilage.

It consists of two components :

1. *Organic material :*
   (a) Collagen : Rich in hydroxyproline
   (b) Ground substance consists of hyaluronic acid.
   (c) Osteoblasts synthesize collagen, matrix etc.
   (d) Osteocytes cause osteolysis.
   (e) Osteoclast degrade bone, activated by PTH.
2. *Inorganic material :* Mainly hydroxyapatite (98%) and $CaHPO_4$ (2%), readily exchangeable, other minerals Na, Mg, K are also present.

   Bone formation is promoted by GH, Vit.-D, calcitonin, PTH, T3 and T4, Insulin etc.

   Loss of bone while mineral to matrix ratio is maintained is known as osteoporosis and is commonly caused by : Idiopathic type — most common, e.g., post menopausal type and Secondary type — caused by excess corticoid hormones etc. Plasma Calcium Phosphorus and alkaline phosphatase levels are normal. It causes spontaneous fractures and morbidity. It can be prevented by physical activity, oestrogen, and adequate Calcium intake.

ADERNAL GLANDS

Medulla

The medulla represents a specialised sympathetic ganglion; it constitutes 25% of the adrenal gland and is surrounded by the cortex. 20% of cells contain no methyltransferase and produce noradrenaline. 80% of cells contain methytransferase which converts noradrenaline to adrenaline. Both cell types produce dopamine which is not released but concerted to noradrenaline.

Preganglionic sympathetic fibres from spinal cord release neurotransmitter acetylcholine on medulla cells. Post ganglionic nerve fibres replace by adrenaline and noradrenaline.

Adrenaline and Noraderaline : Its functions include secretion of adrenaline, noradrenaline and dopamine.

Adrenaline and noradrenaline are derivative of amino acid tyrosine.

Biosynthesis : Tyrosine → Dopa → Dopamine → Noradrenaline → Adrenaline. Their secretion is controlled by preganglionic sympathetic fibres. Stress, angiotensin etc. promote release of adrenaline and noradrenaline.

Mode of action : Adrenaline, noradrenaline and dopamine act through various specific receptors.

1. α Receptors : High affinity for noradenaline.
2. β Receptors : High affinity for adrenaline.
3. γ Receptors : Dominant in vascular smooth muscles etc.
4. D Receptors : High affinity for dopamine. Most abundant in CNS.
5. Receptor populations differ widely from organ to organ.
6. Many drugs affect cellular activity via the adrenergic and dopaminergic receptors.

Their actions include activation of reticular system : Irritability, anxiety etc. In CVS, they accelerate depolarisation of SA node, increase conduction velocity, increase cardiac contractility and irritability, cause vasoconstriction, increase BP. Noradrenaline is more potent hypertensive than adrendine.

Adrenaline dilates eye pupils, relaxes bronchial muscle and is anti-asthmatic. Both adrenaline and noradrenaline increase spinchter tone in GIT and bladder.

Metabolic effects include elevation of blood glucose level, increased glycogenolysis, inhibition of insulin release; it stimulates lipolysis, increases BMR, increases O_2 requirements. Adreanline is more potent than noradrenaline.

Noradrenaline is an important neurotransmitter.

Dopamine

Source : Adrenal medulla and CNS.

Modus operandi

1. Reacts with membrane receptors : D_1 and D_2
2. D_1 present in renal and splanchnic arteries. Both present in some neurons.
3. Its action is centrally as neurotransmitter but unclear peripheral functions.

Pathophysiology : Linked to parkinsonism, huntigton's chorea etc.

Cortex (75%)

It forms outer part of adrenal. It is composed of three layers of epithelial cells: Glomerulosa, Fasciculata, Reticularis.

Cells are rich in cholesterol and Vitamin-C. They synthesize steroid hormones from cholesterol.

Control : Structural and functional integrity regulated by corticotropin.

Chemistry of Corticosteroids : Each hormone possesses the 4-ring steriod nucleus. A double bond is present between C_4 and C_5 of a ring. A CH_3 group is present at C_{10} and C_{13} except in aldosterone. In aldosterone, an aldehye group replaces the methyl group at C_{13}. Functionally, cortico-steroids are subdivided into glucocarticoids, mineralocorticoids and sex hormones. Function of cortical sex hormones (Gonadotropins) is unclear.

Glucocorticoids :

Source : Zona fasciculata and zona reticularis.

Principal glucocorticoid is cortisol (Hydrocortisone) with a half life of 90-100 minutes.

Secretory control regulated by corticotropin from adenohypophysis t½ = 15-25 min.

Corticotropin is regulated by :

1. Cortico liberin
2. Negative feedback by cortisol.

Modus operandi :

1. Hormone combines with cytoplasmic receptors to from a complex.
3. Hormone receptor complex activated and trans-located to nucleus.
4. Hormone reacts with a nucleus receptor and increases mesenger RNA synthesis.
5. Protein synthesis is stimulated.

Actions include stimulated gluconeogenesis from protein; exerts anti-insulin effect and thus cause diabetes; elevates blood glucose level in carbohydrate metabolism.

In protein metabolism they promote proteolysis in skin, bone and muscle and promote gluconeogenesis from amino acids.

In fat metabolism, they stimulate both lipolysis and lipogenesis and promote redistribution of fat.

In vascular system: Condition smooth muscle to adrenaline and noradrenaline.

Muscle activity :

1. *Excess causes proteolysis* : Muscle weak.
2. *Deficiency* : Poor muscle perfusion.

Both excess and deficiency derange nervous function.

In digestive system, stimulate HCl secretion and inhibits cell proliferation in GI tract.

In hemopoietic system, decreases number of circulating eosinophils; decreases lymmocyte population, (increases neutrophils, platelets and red cells).

Inhibits inflammation and allergic reactions by suppressing proteolytic enzymes, capillary permeability, lymphocyte migration and by stabilising membranes. Excessive glucocorticoid inhibits healing.

Regulation of Aldosterone secretion by Renin-Angiotensin Aldosteral (RAA) pathway

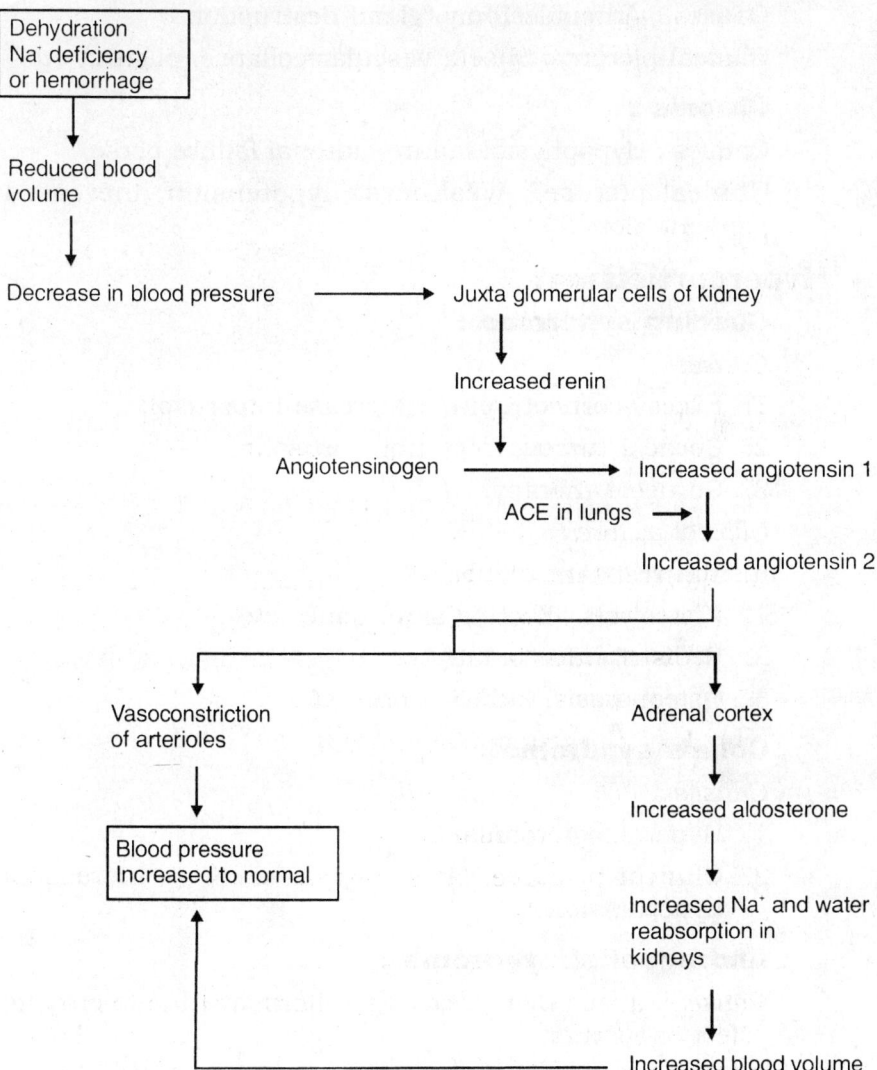

Mineralocorticoids :

Source : Zona glomerulosa – Cells contains 18 aldolase. Principal hormone : Aldosterone; synthesis is aldolase dependent, t ½ = 30 min. The only corticoid with aldehyde at C_{13}. Secretion is stimulated by corticotropin, A II, decreased Na^+ etc.

Modus operandi similar to glucocorticoids; it promotes reabsorption of Na^+ by distal renal tubules and promotes excretion of Na^+ and H^+ by distal tubules.

Hypocorticism :

Acute :
Causes : Adrenalectomy, gland destruction.

Clinical picture : Shock, vascular collapse, oliguria etc.

Chronic :
Causes : Hypophysial failure, adrenal failure perse.

Clinical picture : Weakness, hypotension, increased pigmentation.

Hypercorticism :

Cushing syndrome :
Causes :
1. Excess corticotropin → Increase in cortisol.
2. Cortical tumuor secreting cortisol.
3. Corticoid therapy.

Clinical picture :

Insulin resistant diabetes.
1. Proteolysis affecting skin, bones etc.
2. Redistribution of fat.
3. Osteoporosis, kidney stones etc.

Conn's syndrome :
Causes :
1. Hyperaldosteronism.
2. Clinical picture: Na^+ is increased; K^+ is increased; hypertension.

Androgenital syndrome :
Cause : Caused by increased sex hormone due to enzyme defect or tumuor.

Clinical picture : Virilisation of girls and precocity of boys.

ISLETS OF LANGERHANS

Insulin and glucagon

The islets constitute 2% of the pancreatic mass. It contains four types of cells :
1. A cells : synthesise glucagon.
2. B cells : synthesise insulin.
3. D cells : Synthesise somatostatin.
4. Other type of cells are also present.

Insulin

Its source is B-cells of islets of langerhans. It is produced in thee steps as : preproinsulin – Proinsulin – active insulin.

Proinsulin : It consists of three polypeptides or chains A, B and C. A chain consists of 21 amino acids; B chain contains 30 amino acids; C chain contains 31 amino acids and connects A and B chains.

Active insulin : It contains only A and B chains. C chain is removed before insulin is secreted. An increased level of blood glucose, blood amino acids, blood fatty acids, blood ketone bodies, gastrin, secretin, GIP, GH and CCK, increase insulin secretion. While somatostatin and adrenaline inhibit secretion of insulin, gastrin and secretin. Modus operandi of insulin is that it activates a membrane receptor composed of four chains 2α and 2β. Receptor and insulin complex is internalised by endocytosis.

The effect of insulin on carbohydrate metabolism is that it increases transmembrane transport of glucose in muscle and fat cells, increased metabolism of glucose increases glycogenesis in liver, muscle and fat cells. On fat metabolism is that it increases lipogenesis in fat cells and decreases lipolysis in fat cells. On protein metabolism is that it increases protein synthesis and decreases protein metabolism, increases trans-membrane transport of amino acids, increases growth and spares protein for the body. On potassium metabolism, it increases potassium uptake by cells and hypoinsulism is associated with potassium loss. The hyper-glycaemic hormones like glucocorticoids increase glycogenolysis and decrease glucose metabolism; glucagon increases glycogenolysis in liver and muscle; also increases lipolysis. While growth hormone exhausts β cells and diabetes develops.

Hypoglycaemic hormone is insulin.

Glucagon

Its source is α cells of islets, mucosal cells of stomach and intestine (enteroglucagon). Decrease in plasma glucose stimulates its secretion, increase in plasma amino acids stimulates secretion. Cholecystokinin and gastrin, exercise, stimulate secretion. Somatostatin, secretin, fatty acids and hyperglycaemia inhibit release. Glucagon stimulates glycogenolysis and gluconeogenesis in the liver, stimulates lipolysis in fat cells and plasma fatty acids increase, stimulates proteolysis – gluconeogenesis.

Hypoinsulinism (Diabetes Mellitus)

It is of 3 types :

1. *Junenile onset/type-I/insulin dependent diabetes* : Its onset usually occurs in childhood or in young persons. Onset is abrupt and insulin deficiency is absolute. Patients are usually underweight, hyper-glycaemic, glycosuric and acidotic. Islet cell antibodies are common and patients require insulin therapy.
2. *Maturity onset/type-II/Insulin independent diabetes* : It occurs chiefly in later life. Genetic factor common. It comes on gradually and patients are mostly obese, hyperglycaemic and glycosuric; acidosis is uncommon. Plasma insulin level may be low, normal or high. It is managed by dietary regimen and oral hypoglycemic therapy.
3. *Secondary onset diabetes* : Its onset is secondary to excess glucocorticoids, GH, etc. Acidosis is un-common. Plasma insulin level is normal, and is strikingly insulin resistant.

Hyperinsulinism

It may result from insulin therapy, insulin secreting tumour etc. It is characterised by mental confusion and decreased muscle tone, locomotion disturbances, low plasma glucose and insulin levels, coma and death.

AGING AND THE ENDOCRINE SYSTEM

1. Some endocrine glands shrink in size with age but their activity may or may not be reduced.
2. Production of some hormones is reduced with age — growth hormone, thyroid hormones, cortisol, aldosterone, estrogens.
3. Levels of some hormones are raised with age – TSH, LH, FSH and PTH.
4. Release of insulin reduces with age and also receptor sensitivity to glucose decreases.
5. Size of the thymus begins to decrease with age after puberty.

16

REPRODUCTION

INTRODUCTION

All organ systems of body operate as homeostatic controls to maintain the psychophysiological wellbeing of the individual. At the organization level, reproduction may be regarded as a homeostatic control adopted for survival of the species.

MALE REPRODUCTIVE SYSTEM

Reproductive system organs may be classified as :

Essential organs — For production of gametes.

Accessory organs — Play supportive role in the reproductive process.

In both sexes the essential organs for reproduction that produce the gametes or sex cells are called gonads.

Male gonads are the testes, the accessory organs are genital tracts, glands and supportive structures.

Accessory glands in the reproductive system produce secretions that serve to nourish, transport and mature sperms. The glands are a pair of seminal vesicle, one prostate and a pair of Cowper's glands.

The supporting structures are scrotum, penis and a pair of spermatic cords.

Functions of Male Reproductive System

1. Testes — Produces sperms and the male sex hormone - testosterone.
2. Ducts — Transport, store and assist in maturation of sperm.
3. Accessory sex glands — Secrete most of the liquid portion of semen.
4. Penis — It contains urethra and it serves as an organ of copulation and ejaculation of semen. It is also a passage way for urine excretion.

Structure	Function
Testis	Produce sperms and sex hormone

Accessory organs
  Scrotum
  Penis
  Vas deferens
  Seminal vesicles
  Cowper's gland
  Prostrate
	
	Houses the testis
	Organ of copulation and excretion
	Carry sperm out of the body
	Majority of fluid within semen

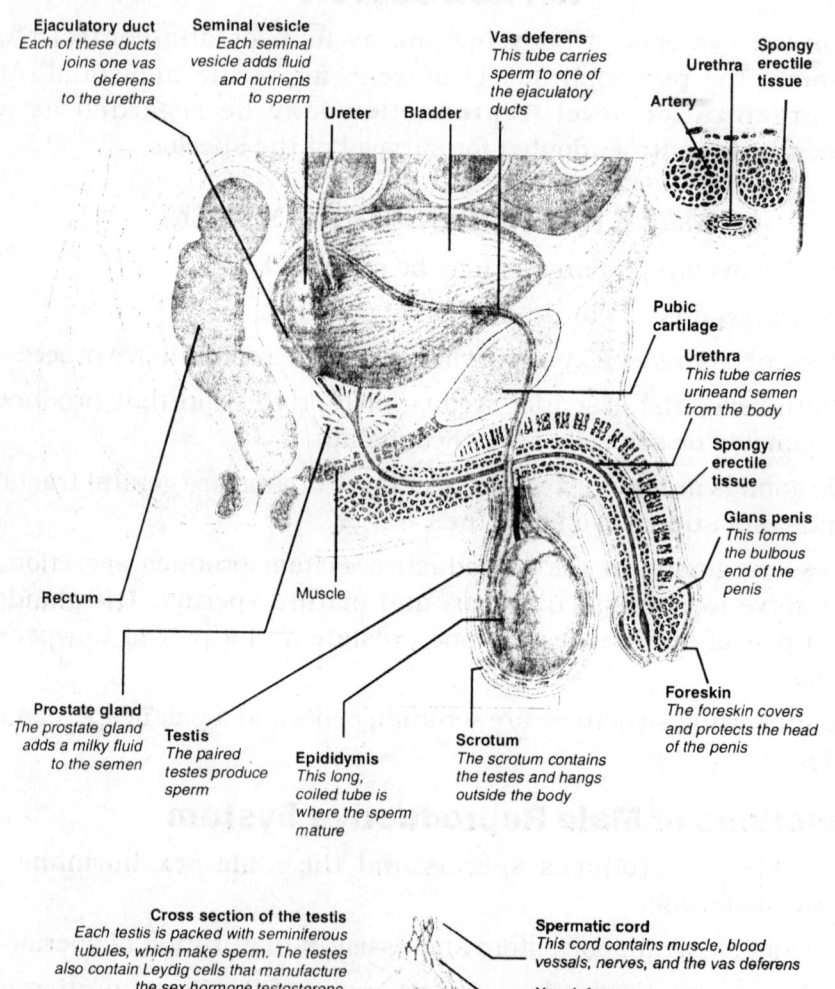

Fig. 16.1 Male reproductive system.

Function of testes

Testes has two primary functions — spermatogenesis and secretion of hormones.

Supermatogenesis : It is the production of sperm. Seminiferous tubules produce the sperm. It involves mitosis, meiosis and a process called spermiogenesis.

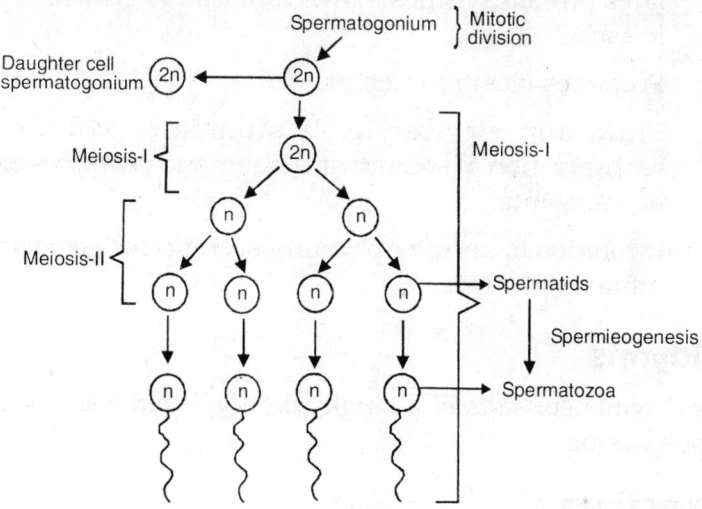

Fig. 16.2 Spermatogenesis.

The above flow chart shows how a single spermatogonium gives rise to four spermatozoa.

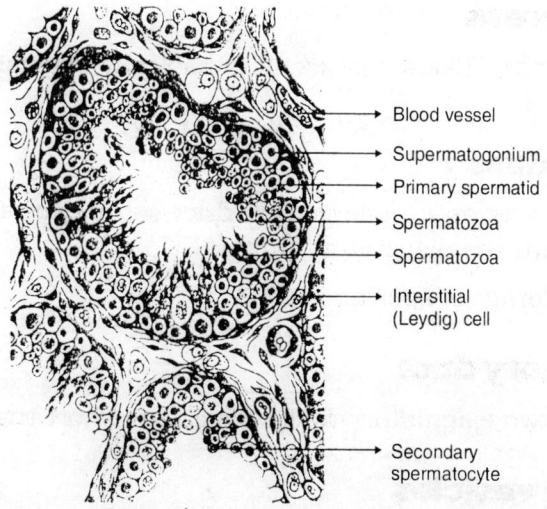

Fig. 16.3 Section of testis showing stages of spermatogenesis.

Hormonal secretion : Mainly testosterone is secreted by Leydig cells. Testosteron; plays following functions :

1. Promotes the development of male secondary sex characteristics, accessory organs such as pro-state, seminal vesicles etc.
2. It is a anabolic hormone it regulates metabolism, it stimulates protein synthesis therefore lead to growth of skeletal muscle.
3. Promotes closure of epiphysis.
4. Fluid and electrolyte. It stimulates kidney tubule reabsorp-tion of sodium and water and promotes excretion of potassium.
5. Inhibition of anterior pituitary secretion of gon-adotropins named FSH, LH.

Epididymis

Each epidymis consists of a single, tightly coiled tube enclosed in a fibrous casing.

Functions :
1. It has the function of sperm passage from testis to exterior.
2. It secretes small amount of seminal fluid.
3. Maturation of sperms.

Vas deferens

It is also a tube like structure. It is basically extension epididymis tail.

Functions :
1. It acts as a male genital duct connecting the epididymis with the ejaculatory duct.
2. Storage of sperm.

Ejaculatory duct

There are two ejaculatory ducts which are short tube like.

Seminal vesicles

These are convoluted pouches that lie along the lower part of posterior surface of the bladder.

Functions : It secretes an alkaline, viscous liquid to the semen. This helps in protection of sperms from acid in the male urethra and female vagina.

Prostate

It is a tubuloalveolar gland lying below the bladder.

Functions : It secretes a thin alkaline substance that contributes to the seminal fluid. This alkalinity helps to protect the sperm from acid in the male urethra and female vagina and increases sperm motility.

Cowpers gland

It acts like prostate; it secretes an alkaline fluid that increases sperm motility by protecting them from acid.

FEMALE REPRODUCTIVE SYSTEM

Female reproductive system is important for production of offspring and existence of genetic code.

The female reproductive system provides nutrition and protection to the developing offspring for upto several years after conception.

The primary sex organs are the paired ovaries which produce oocyte and also contain endocrine cells which produce and secrete the hormones progesteron, oestrogen and relaxin.

The accessary reproductive organs consist of fallopian tube, the uterus and the external genitalia.

Structure	Function
Ovaries	Produce ova and sex hormones.
Fallopian tube	Carry ova from ovary to uterus.
Vagina	Receive sperm during intercourse.
Vulva	Protection.
Uterus	Nourishes development of embryo.

Ovaries

The paired ovaries are structure about twice the size of almond nuts. They are supported by ovarian ligaments, suspensory ligaments which anchor them to pelvic cavity.

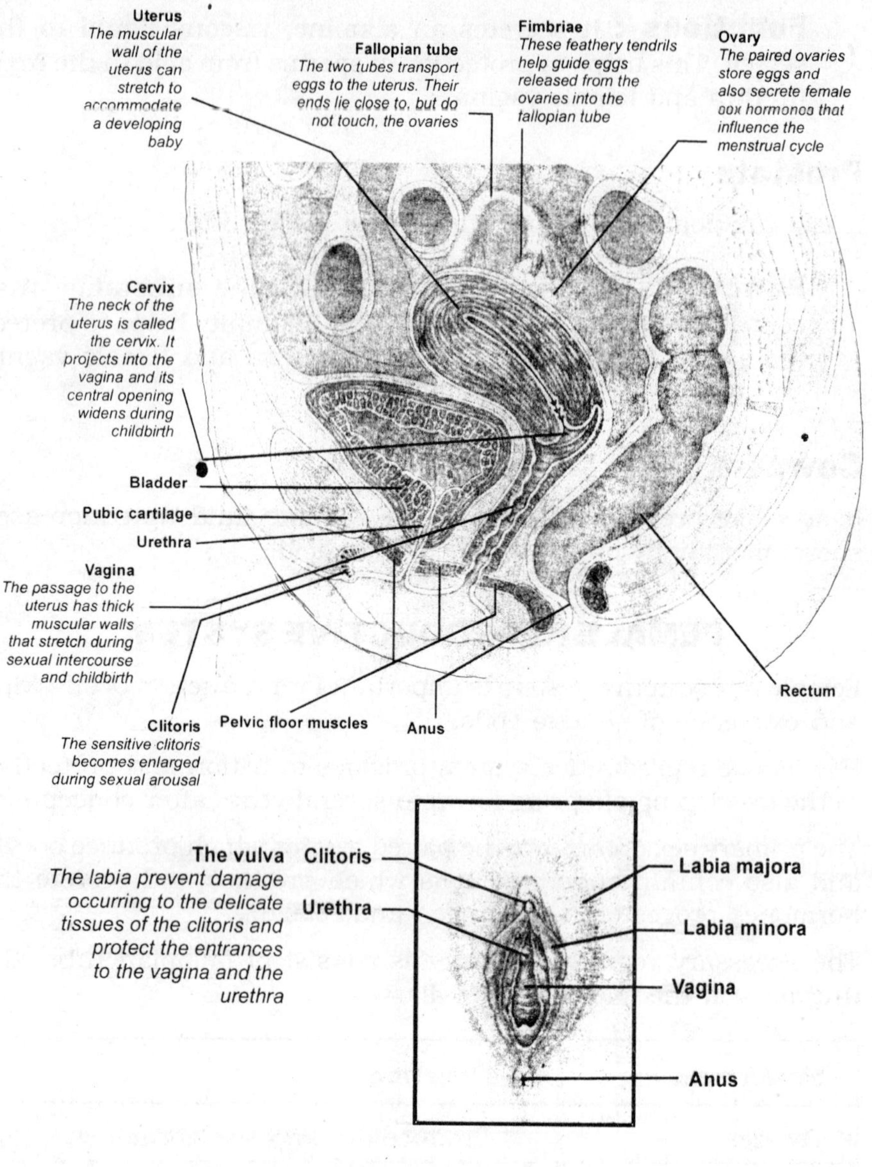

Fig. 16.4 Female reproductive system.

Ovaries' cortex contains ovarian follicles. Each follicle consists of an immature egg. As the menstural cycle proceeds, the follicles progressively change their structure as following :

Primary follicle

↓

Secondary follicle

↓

Graffian follicle
↓
Corpus luteum

Fallopian tubes

They transport the secondary oocyte, if fertilization has taken place, to the uterus. Each tube is 10 cm long and has an isthmus, ampulla and the infundibulum as shown in the following diagram:

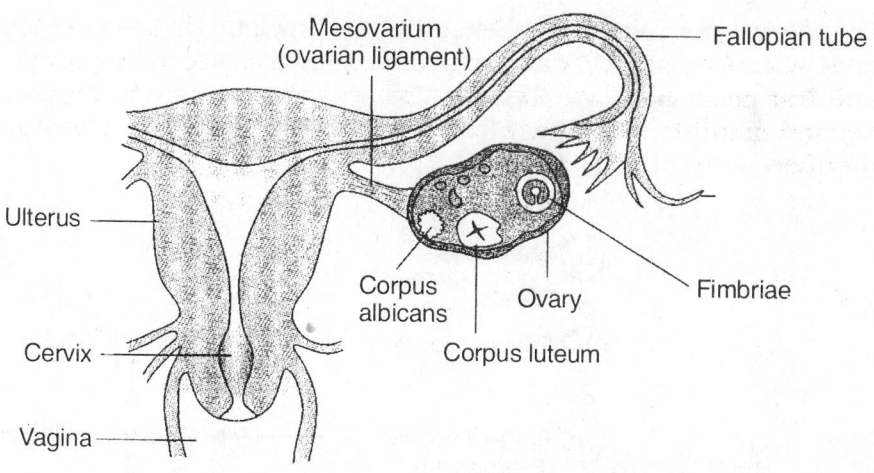

Fig. 16.5 The Female genital tract.

Uterus

It is located between the bladder and the rectum. It is the site of menstruation, implantation, embryo-fetal development and labour.

Vagina

It is a thin walled, muscular, tubular organ lying between the urinary bladder and the rectum and extends from cervix to the external genital opening.

Vagina conveys uterine secretions to outside of body, receives erect penis during sexual intercourse, and transports fetus during its birth.

Oogenesis

It is female homologue of spermatogenesis. Oogonium are the stem cells which after first meiotic division produce the primary oocyte.

The below diagram clearly illustrates the oogenesis. The female oogonia which is diploid multiply by mitosis to produce reserve germ cells. Then oogonia enters growth phase and primor-dial follicle appears and oogonia are converted to primary oocyte. Primary follicle develops from primordial follicle and then growing follicle and graffican follicle finally converting to ovulated secondary oocyte.

In their life a female supplies 7,50,000 of primary oocyte. These cells are stalled in the early stages of the first meiotic division and will not complete meiosis unless stimulated by hormonal changes after puberty.

One oocyte per month completes the first meiotic division, which ends when two haploid daughters cells known as secondary oocyte and first polar body are formed. The secondary oocyte undergoes second meiotic division after fertilization and this division produces second polar body.

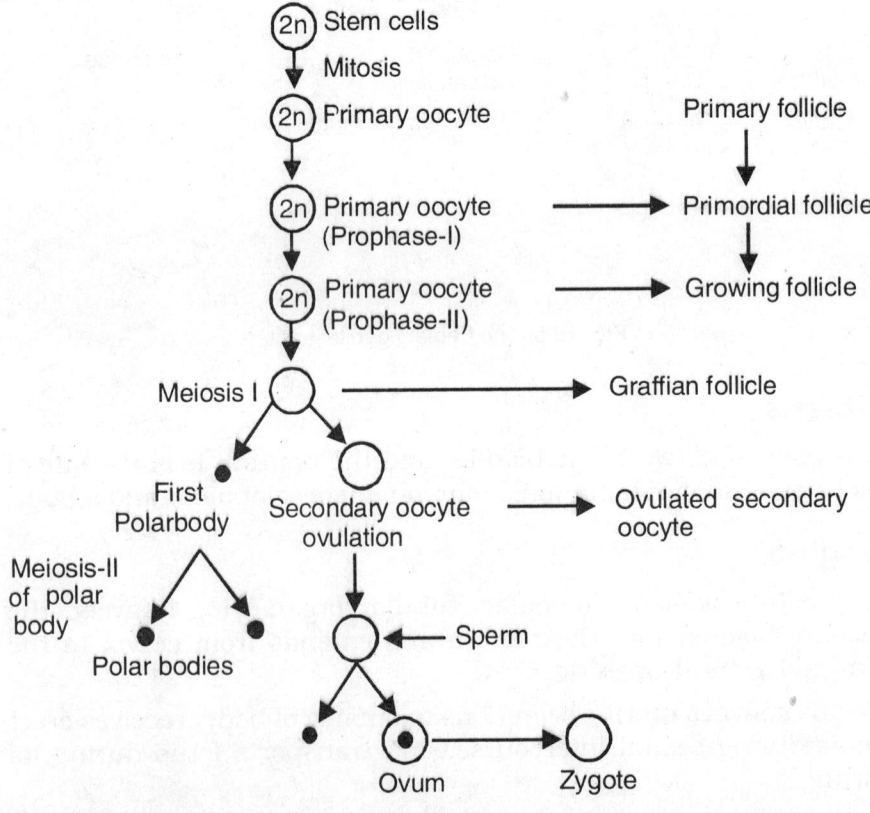

Fig. 16.6 Oogenesis.

Menstural cycle

The compact and spongy layers of the endometrium slough off during menstrual cycle.

The organs primarily affected are ovaries, uterus and vagina.

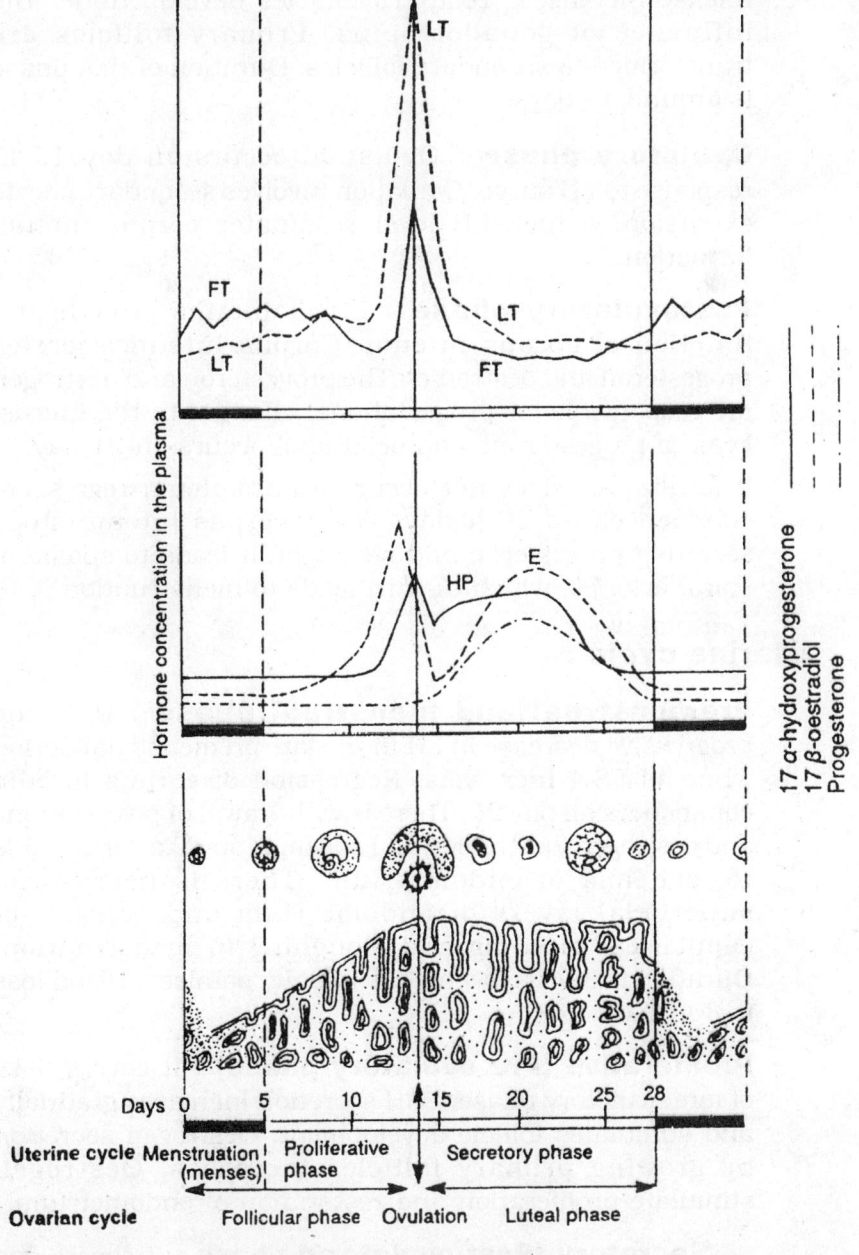

Fig. 16.7 The menstrual cycle.

Ovarian cycle :

1. Preovulatory phase
2. Ovulatory phase
3. Postovulatory phase

Preovulatory phase : In this phase gonadotropin release increases, 10 to 15 follicles develop under the influence of gonadotropins. Primary follicles are transformed to secondary follicles. Duration of this phase is around 14 days.

Ovulatory phase : Ovulation occurs on day 15 in response to LH surge. Ovulation involves secondary oocyte extrusion. A high LH level stimulates corpus luteum formation.

Postovulatory phase : LH maintains growth and function of corpus luteum. Corpus luteum secretes progesteron and oestradiol. The progesteron and oestrogen are responsible for progestational changes in the uterus. Peak of progesterone and oestradiol occurs on 21 day.

If fertilization does not occur corpus luteum regression commences on 26th day. When corpus luteum stops secreting progesteron and oestrogen it leads to spasm of spiral arteries, which in turn leads to menstruation.

Uterine cycle :

Premenstrual and menstrual phase : It is the progressive decrease in LH in the late premenstrual period whereas FSH increases. Regression of corpus luteum commences on day 26. There is withdrawal of progesterone and oestrogen (oestradiol) and spasm of spiral arteries leads to ischemia of endometrium. There is necrosis of superficial layers of endometrium and rupture of capillaries, bleeding and sloughing in menstruation. Duration is 3-7 days which is usually painless. Blood loss is 30-50 ml.

Proliferative (Pre ovulatory phase) : It covers 3-14 of fore ovuletory phase. FSH secretion increases gradually and stimulates follicle development. Oestrogen secretion by growing primary follicles increases. Oestrogen stimulate proliferation and restoration of endometrium.

Secretory (Post ovulatory) phase : It covers day 15-28. Initially FSH and LH levels are fairly high.

Progesterone and oestradiol levels peak on day 21. Deep parts of uterine glands dilate and secretory activity increases. Decidual cells stores nutrients. LH and FSH levels decrease due to negative feedback. Regression commences resulting in progesterone and estrogen withdrawal. Spasm of spiral arteries causes vasodilatation and menstrual stage commences.

Vaginal cycle : Oestrogen stage (days 13-14) — cornification of vaginal epithelium and glucose increase. Progesterone stage (days 16-27) — maturation, desquamation and clumping of epithelium, glucose decreases, leukocyte infiltraton occurs.

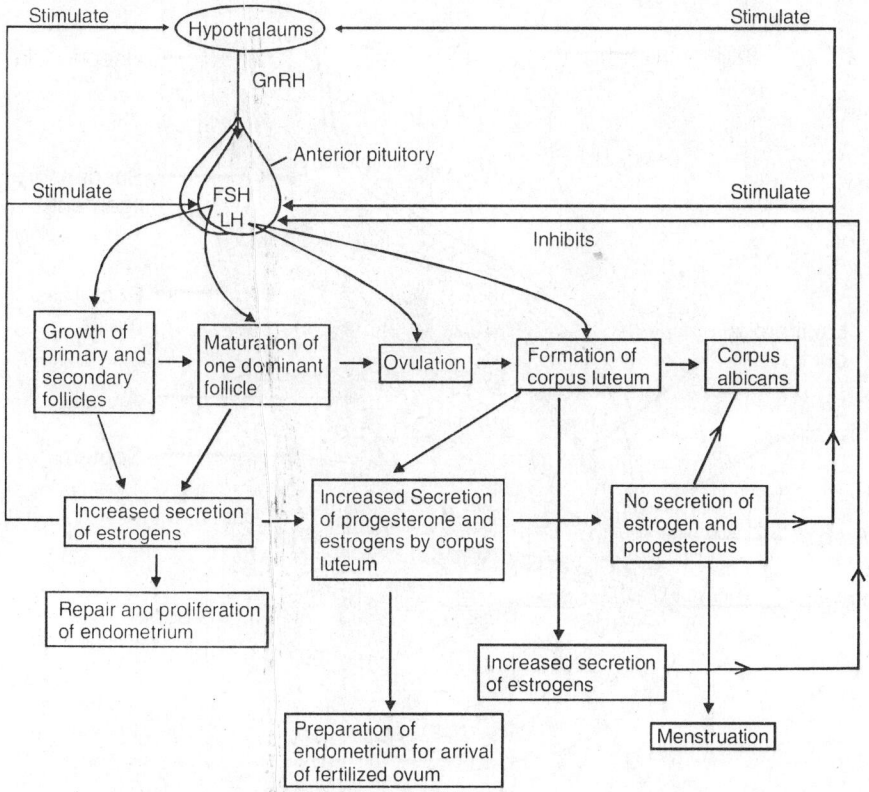

Fig. 16.8 Hormonal interactions in the ovarion and uterine cycles.

THE BREAST

The breasts overlie the pectoral muscles and are attached to them by a layer of connective tissue. Breast development is controlled by two hormones — oestrogen and progesterone.

Estrogen

It stimulates growth of the ducts of mammary glands.

Progesterone

It stimulate development of actual secreting cells.

Each breast is made up of several lobes separated by septa of connective tissue. Each lobe consists of several lobules, which are made of connective tissue in which the alveoli are embedded. The ducts from the various lobules unite to form a single lactiferous duct for each lobe.

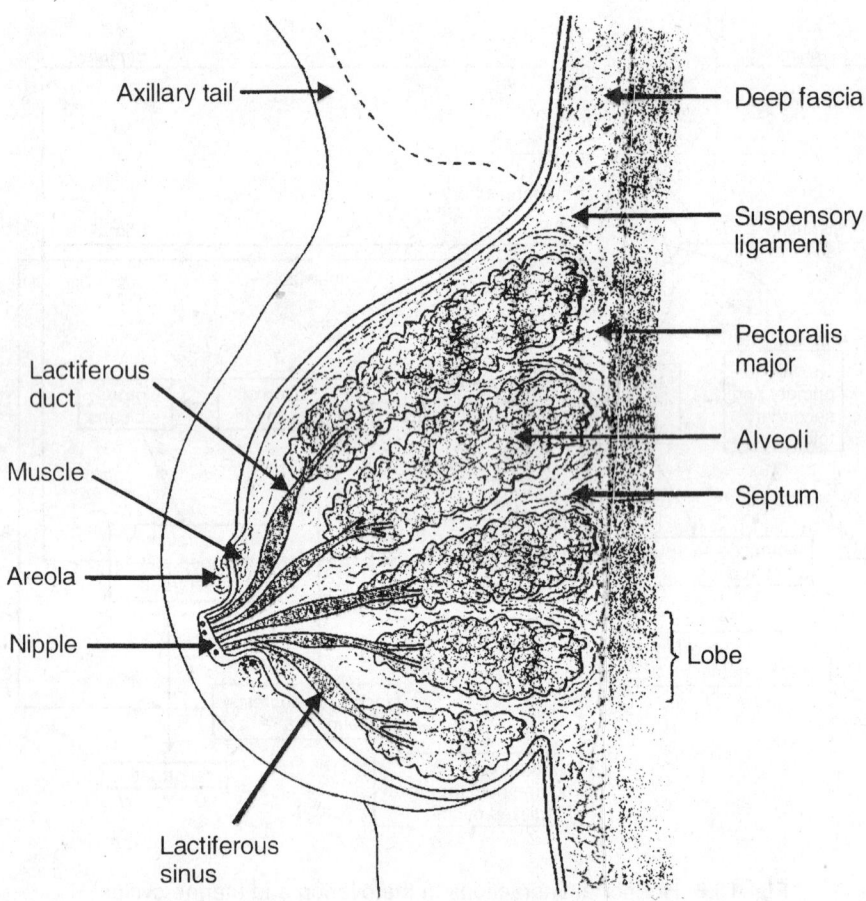

Fig. 16.9 The female breast.

Areola

The nipples are bordered by a circular pigmented area. It contains numerous sebaceous glands that appear as small nodules under the skin.

Lactation

The main function of mammary glands is lactation. Lactation means secretion of milk.

Mechanism of lactation : The given flow chart illustrates the mechanism controlling lactation:

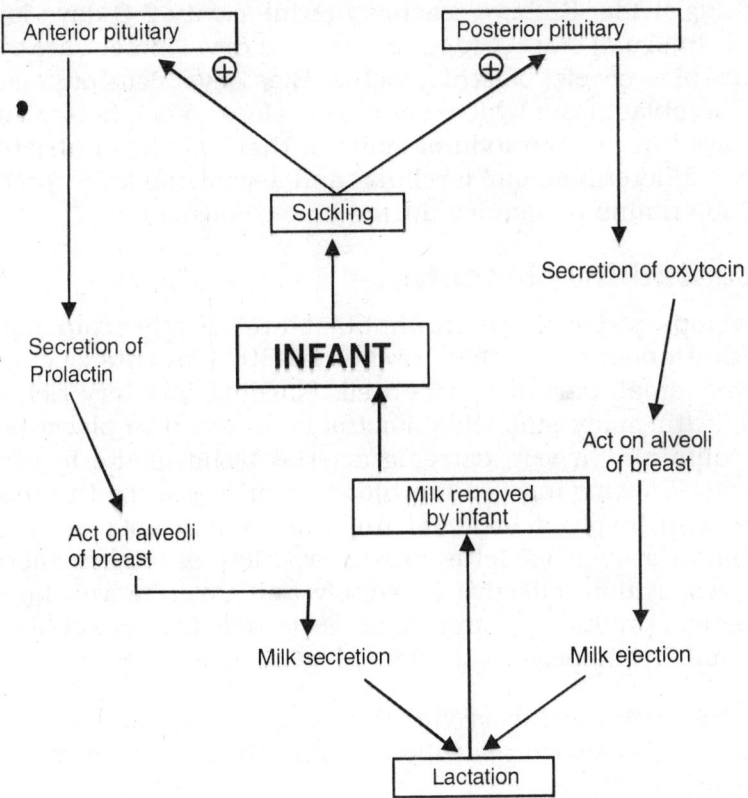

The above flow chart shows how the infant is able to take milk from the breast of her mother. During lactation main action of suckling stimulates secretions from anterior and posterior pituitary glands finally leading to secretion and ejection of milk from the female breast.

Mother milk is best for the nourishment of the infant because :

1. It has rich amount of proteins, fat, vitamins, calcium.
2. It provides passive immunity to offspring because the mother's milk contains antibodies.
3. It helps in development of jaw of the infant.
4. It protects the infant from several diseases.
5. It acts as an emotional bond between mother and the child.

EMBRYOGENESIS

Fertilisation / implantation

Fertilisation occurs in uterine tube and fertilised ovum (zygote) begins to divide. Embryo reaches uterine cavity 2-3 days later at 16 cells (morula) stage. Stages in prenatal development are zygote, morula, blastocoele, blastula, foetus. Blastocyst cells organised in an embryoblast from which embryo develops; a trophoblast which is involved in implantation of embryo, that supplies nutrients for embryo, differentiate into a cellular and a syncytial layer, produces HCG, maintains pregnancy during first trimester.

Placentation / placenta

It develops partly from trophoblast and partly from mother. Placentation is completed by day 70-90. Placenta occupies a relatively small part of uterine well. Placenta has very rich blood supply with many sinusoids. Foetus is attached to placenta by a cord containing a vein carrying arterial blood to the foetus and two arteries carrying venous blood from foetus to the mother. Placenta is involved in foetal nutrition which acts as nutrient absorption system for fetus, waste products of fetal metabolism; foetal respiration, effective O_2 supply and Co_2 removal, hormone production, produces oestrogen, progesterone, fetal protection, acts as ultrafilter and permits transfer of IgG.

Chorion : It forms villi that project into maternal blood sinusoids. Also forms superficial membrane that covers foetus superficially.

Amnion and amnon fluid : Amniotic membrane surrounds foetus immediately and contains amniotic fluid. Amniotic fluid volume is 500-1000 ml and contains protein and glucose, etc. Amniotic fluid serves as protective shock absorber for foetus, permits free movements of fetus and amniocentesis provides valuable clinical information.

Hydramnios is excessive amnion fluid formation. Rupture of chorion and amnion and escape of fluid preceeds birth of baby.

HOMOLOGUS STRUCTURES OF MALE AND FEMALE REPRODUCTIVE SYSTEMS

Male Structure	Female Sturcture
1. Testes	1. Ovaries
2. Spermatozoa	2. Ovum
3. Scrotum	3. Lobia majora
4. Penile urethra	4. Lobia minora
5. Membranous urethra	5. Vestibule
6. Corpus spongiosum of penis	6. Bulb of vestibule
7. Glans penis	7. Clitoris
8. Prostate	8. Paraurethral glands
9. Cowper's glands	9. Greater vestibular glands

**PUNCTUALITY IS
THE SOUL OF ALL BUSINESSES.**

IMPORTANT QUESTIONS

BIOCHEMICAL AND BIOPHYSICAL PRINCIPLE

Written exam

1. Role of transport mechanisms
2. Osmosis
3. Diffusion
4. Active vs passive transport
5. Secondary active transport
6. Transportation process
7. Equivalents
8. Dialysis
9. Homeostasis
10. $Na^+ - K^+$ pump
11. Principle of receptors
12. Active transport mechanism
13. Exocytosis and endocytosis
14. Electrolyte concentration of plasma and urine
15. Facultative transport
16. Principle ways of chemical messengers

Viva

- Transport mechanism
- Dialysis
- What is physiology
- Exo and endocytosis

NUTRITION AND HEALTH

Written exam

1. Define nutrition
2. What is metabolism
3. Define role of proteins, carbohydrates and fat
4. Milk (mothers)
5. Short note on uses of nutrients
6. What are major and minor nutrients
7. What happens when digestion of carbohydrate occurs in the body.

Viva

- Anabolism
- Catabolism
- Clinical uses of nutrients
- Balanced diet
- Major nutrients
- Micro nutrients

THE BLOOD

Written exam

1. What are the different constituents of blood.
2. Eosinophils (diag) and functions.
3. Monocyte.
4. Eosinophilia.
5. Rh incompatibility.
6. Rh factor.
7. Illustrate with the help of diagram the commonest type of leucocytes.
8. Polymorphonuclear cells.
9. Intrinsic pathway.
10. Extrinsic pathway.
11. Platelets.
12. How platelet plug is formed.
13. Prothrombin time.
14. What is anaemia.
15. The plasma.
16. Haemoglobin.
17. Plama vs serum.
18. What is fetal and adult Hb.

RETICULOENDOTHEUAL SYSTEM

Written exam

1. Function of lymph.
2. Spleen.
3. What is meant by reticuloendothelial system.

Viva
- Lymph.
- Role of reticuloendothelial system.
- Spleen role in immunity.
- Lymphatic regulation.
- Role of lymph node.

CARDIOVASCULAR SYSTEM

Written exam
1. Triple response.
2. Blood pressure.
3. Factors affecting blood pressure.
4. Discuss the regulation of B.P.
5. Radial pulse.
6. Changes in coronary blood flow.
7. Cardiac impulse.
8. Regulation of blood.
9. Special features of pulmonary circulation.
10. Describe special features and regulation of blood flow to:
    (a) Brain
    (b) Skin
11. ECG.
12. Cyanosis.
13. What is meant by shock?
14. What are different types of shock?
15. Baroreceptors.
16. Apex beat.
17. State the law of starling.

Viva
- Blood pressure and its regulation.
- Apex beat.
- Regional circulation.
- ECG.
- Brain circulation.
- CSF
- BBB (Blood Brain Barrier)
- Role of circulation
- Blood constituent

RESPIRATION

Written exam
1. Anatomy and physiology of respiratory organs.
2. FEV.
3. The non-respiratory functions of lungs.
4. Tidal volume
5. Vital capacity
6. Regulation of respiration.
7. Functional capacity
8. Normal spirogram
9. What is surfactant
10. Neural regulation of respiration
11. FEV_1, FEV_2, FEV_3
12. Spirometry
13. Draw a normal spirogram
14. Carbon dioxide transport
15. Ventilation perfusion
16. O_2 and CO_2 transport
17. Short note on haldane effect
18. Bohr effect
19. Describe effect of high altitude on respiration.
20. Dyspnoea
21. Hypoxia
22. Respiratory membrane.
23. Neural regulation of respiration.

Viva
- Spirometery
- Hypoxia
- Dyspnoea
- Apnoea
- Artificial respiration
- Respiratory membrane
- Bohr effect
- Haldane effect
- CO_2 and O_2 transport

KIDNEY

Written exam
1. Nephron

2. Cortical and J.M. Nephron
3. Anatomy and physiology of kidney
4. G.F.R.
5. Blood circulation in kidney
6. Juxta-glomerular apparatus
7. Filtration regulation
8. Transport maximum
9. Micturition
10. Urine formation
11. Clearance
12. Electrolyte transport
13. Factors affecting G.F.R.
14. Glomerulotubular balance.
15. Describe briefly the regulation of glumerulo-filtration rate

Viva
- Functional unit of kidney
- Electrolyte transport
- Urine formation
- Role of kidney in urine formation.

NERVOUS SYSTEM
Written exam
1. Synapse
2. Type of synapse
3. Draw labelled diag. of vestibular apparatus.
4. Reflex
5. Brain connection.
6. Basal ganglia
7. Receptors
8. Vestibular apparatus
9. How is body posture maintained
10. Describe the circulation and functions of C.S.F.
11. Pain
12. EEG.
13. Basal ganglia functions
14. Cerebellum role
15. Role of hypothalamus

Viva
- Reflex arc
- Receptors
- Synapse
- Role of cerebellum

SPECIAL SENSES
Written exam
1. Accommodation
2. Error of refractions
3. Direct light reflex
4. Myopia
5. Hypermetropia
6. Pathway of consensual reflex
7. Dark adaptation
8. Draw diag. of retina
9. Light reflex
10. Role of rods and cones in colour vision
11. Function of cochlea
12. Organ of corti
13. Role of middle ear in hearing
14. Malingering
15. Olfactory pathway
16. Taste pathway

Viva
- Accommodation
- Refractive errors
- Rods and cones
- Layers of retina

DIGESTIVE SYSTEM
Written exam
1. What happens and why to digestion of fat
2. Protein digestion
3. Peristalsis
4. Biological value of protein.
5. Vomiting mechanism
6. Gastro - intestinal hormones
7. Gastrin
8. Liver salts

9. Major functions of small intestines
10. Entero - Hepatic circulation of salt
11. Bile functions and contents
12. Saliva
13. Salivary gland
14. Digestion
15. Digestive organs.

Viva
- GIT hormones
- Entero-hepatic circulation
- Role of peristalsis
- Peristalsis
- Liver salts
- Role of bile salts
- Nutrition
- Constituents of saliva

INTEGUMENTARY SYSTEM

Written exam
1. Role of skin
2. Skin glands
3. Temperature regulation by skin.

Viva
- Skin glands.
- Role of skin.

HORMONES (ENDOCRINE)

Written exam
1. Anterior pituitary hormones
2. Proinsulin
3. Insulin
4. Thyroid hormones
5. Glucagon
6. Hormonal cycle
7. Post-pituitary hormones
8. Various ways of hormonal actions
9. GIT hormones
10. Hypoglycemia
11. Pancreatic hormones

Viva
- What are hormones
- Ant. pituitary hormones
- Post. pituitary hormones
- Insulin

REPRODUCTIVE SYSTEM

Written exam
1. Oogenesis
2. Role of menstrual cycle
3. Primary sex organs
4. Ovaries
5. Spermiogenesis
6. Sex linked diseases
7. Conception
8. Prostate
9. Hormonal cycle of menstrual period
10. Menopause vs menarche
11. Prime organs of reproduction
12. Why reproduction is essential

Viva
- Spermatogenesis
- Spermiogenesis
- Oogenesis
- Menstrual cycle

MULTIPLE CHOICE QUESTION

Q1. Normal QRS interval is
- a — 0.2 sec.
- b — 0.4 – 0.6 sec.
- c — 0.08 – 0.1 sec.
- d — 1.0 – 1.5 sec.

Ans. c

Q2. Length of distal convoluted tubule is
- a — 2 mm
- b — 5 mm
- c — 8 mm
- d — 12 mm

Ans. b

Q3. In strenous exercise PCO_2 fall from
- a — 40 to 15
- b — 60 to 35
- c — 25 to 10
- d — 35 to 0

Ans. a

Q4. Alkalosis occurs whenever pH is above
- a — 7.00
- b — 7.24
- c — 7.36
- d — 7.40

Ans. d

Q5. Work done in quiet breathing is
- a — 0.1 kg m/min
- b — 0.2 kg m/min
- c — 0.5 kg m/min
- d — 2.5 kg m/min

Ans. c

Q6. Functional residual capacity in male is
- a — 3.8 liters
- b — 3.3 liters
- c — 2.8 liters
- d — 2.2 liters

Ans. d

Q7. In humans effective renal blood flow is
- a — 425
- b — 525
- c — 625
- d — 725

Ans. c

Q8. Blood flow in carotid body in ml/100 gm of tissue
- a — 500
- b — 1000
- c — 2000
- d — 4000

Ans. c

Q9. Bound $1C^+$ is mainly found in following except
- a — Brain
- b — Bone
- c — RBC
- d — Platelets

Ans. d

Q9. Neurotransmitter which controls secretion of prolactin
- a — Serotonin
- b — Gaba
- c — Somatostatin
- d — Dopamine

Ans. c

Q10. Conduction velocity is least in
a — AV node
b — Bundle of his
c — SA node
d — Purkinje fibre

Ans. a

Q11. Broca's area is present in
a — Superior temporal gyrus
b — Precentral gyrus
c — Postcentral gyrus
d — Inferior frontal gyrus

Ans. d

Q12. The ECG curves are called
a — ABCDE curves
b — Berger's curves
c — Neurogenic curves
d — REM rhythm

Ans. a, c, d

Q13. Under resting condition the cardiac output is — l/min.
a — 2.5
b — 4.25
c — 5.25
d — 9.5
e — 7.5

Ans. c

Q14. Spirometery measures except
a — Tidal volume
b — Vital capacity
c — Fev
d — none

Ans. d

Q15. In excitable cell, repolarisation is closely associated with one of the following
a — Na^+ efflux
b — Na^+ influx
c — K^+ efflux
d — K^+ influx

Ans. c

Q16. The EEG rhythm having lowest frequency
a — Alpha
b — Beta
c — Delta
d — Theta

Ans. c

Q17. How many Pka values does orthophosphoric acid possess
a — one
b — two
c — three
d — four

Ans. c

Q18. Venoconstriction is exhibited by all except
a — Valsalva manoeuvre
b — Asphyxia
c — Haemorrhage
d — Lying down

Ans. d

Q19. In female genital tract the spermatozoa do not live more than
a — 12 hrs.
b — 24 hrs.
c — 36 hrs.
d — 48 hrs.

Ans. d

Q20. The diffusing capacity for carbon dioxide compared to that for oxygen

a — 20 times
b — 10 times
c — 5 times
d — 2 times

Ans. a

Q21. Total vital capacity is decreased but timed vital capacity is normal in
a — Bronchial Asthma
b — Scoliosis
c — Chronic bronchitis
d — All the above

Ans. b

Q22. The intrapleural pressure at the end of deep inspiration is
a — − 4 mmHg
b — + 4 mmHg
c — − 16 mmHg
d — + 18 mmHg

Ans. a

Q23. Essential hypertension is generally associated with an early increase in
a — Oxygen
b — Coronary flow
c — Cardiac work
d — Cardiac output

Ans. c

Q24. A procoagulant not normally circulating in plasma is
a — Prothrombin
b — Fibrinogen
c — Antihemophilic factor
d — Factor V
e — None

Ans. e

Q25. The Ionic channel in excitable membrane are lined by
a — Cophalin
b — Protein
c — Lipid
d — Carbohydrates.

Ans. b

Q26. Macrophages are the mature form of
a — Neutrophil
b — Eosinophil
c — Basophil
d — Monocytes
e — Lymphocytes

Ans. d

Q27. Maximum absorption of bile occur at
a — Jejunum
b — Duodenum
c — Illeum
d — Colon

Ans. c

Q28. What is the glomerular filtration rate
a — 100 ml/min
b — 125 ml/min
c — 150 ml/min
d — 175 ml/min
e — 200 ml/min

Ans. b

Q29. Compliance of lung is decreased in all conditions except
a — Fibrosis of lung
b — Emphysema
c — Pulmonary oedema

Ans. b

Q30. Smoking cause
a — Decreased ciliary motility
b — Cellular hyperplasia

c — Mucous secretion
d — All

Ans. d

Q31. The medium with highest refractive index in the eye is
a — Cornea
b — Nucleus of lens
c — Cortex of lens
d — Aqueous

Ans. b

Q32. Blood brain barrier is made up of
a — Astrocytes
b — Oligodendrocytes
c — Oligodendroglia
d — Microglia

Ans. a

Q33. Neutropenia is seen in all except
a — Pernicious anaemia
b — Severe bacterial infection
c — Trauma
d — Bone marrow depression

Ans. c

Q34. Oxygen dissociation curve is
a — Bell shaped
b — S-shaped
c — Normal wave type
d — Delta shaped

Ans. b

Q35. Colour blindness is called
a — Deuteranopia
b — Protanopia
c — Protanomaly
d — Deuteranomaly

Ans. b

Q36. The normal A/G ratio is
a — 5 : 1
b — 2 : 1
c — 1 : 2
d — 1 : 1

Ans. b

Q37. Velocity of blood at normal cardiac output in the aorta is
a — 32 cm/sec.
b — 64 cm/sec.
c — 8 cm/sec.
d — 30 cm/sec.

Ans. a

Q38. Following are the local hormone
a — Insulin
b — Heparin
c — Bradykinin
d — Acetylcholine

Ans. a

Q39. Which one of the following is released by blood platelets during hemorrhage to produce vasoconstriction.
a — Serotonin
b — Histamine
c — Thrombus thenin
d — Bradyikinin

Ans. a

Q40. The most important substance controlling alveolar ventilation.
a — O_2
b — CO_2
c — H_2O
d — None

Ans. b

Q41. An adult human pancrease is about

- a — 100-2000 / slets
- b — 100,000-200,000 / slets
- c — 250,000-750,0000 / slets
- d — above 1000,000 / slets

Ans. c

Q42. Stapes rest in
- a — Round window
- b — Oval window
- c — Tympanic membrane
- d — Basilar membrane

Ans. a

Q43. Peak testosterone level are seen at about
- a — 7-8 p.m.
- b — 2 a.m.
- c — 7-8 a.m.
- d — 12 p.m.

Ans. c

Q44. Heart rate is maximum in normal
- a — Foetus
- b — Newborn
- c — Adult
- d — Old age

Ans. a

Q45. The non ionic diffusion in body is seen in
- a — Gut
- b — Kidney
- c — Both
- d — None

Ans. c

Q46. The band which disappears on muscle contraction is
- a — H
- b — I
- c — A
- d — Z

Ans. a

Q47. The band which appears on muscular contraction is
- a — Z
- b — A
- c — I
- d — M or cm

Ans. c

Q48. The excretion of sodium in 24 hrs.
- a — 0
- b — 50
- c — 150
- d — 250

Ans. c

Q49. Gag reflex is mediated by cranial nerve
- a — vi
- b — ix
- c — x
- d — xii

Ans. b

Q50. The renal blood flow is
- a — 250
- b — 800
- c — 1260
- d — 1500

Ans. c

Q51. Bath motropic effect is produced by
- a — Stimulation of vagus
- b — Nerve other than vagus
- c — Atropine
- d — Section of vagus

Ans. a

Q52. The alveolar PO$_2$ is
  a — 100 mmHg
  b — 110 mmHg
  c — 120 mmHg
  d — 150 mmHg
Ans. a

Q53. All are seen in obesity except
  a — Diabetes
  b — Hyperuricemia
  c — Atherosclerosis
  d — Increased sensitivity to GH
Ans. d

Q54. Normal functional residual capacity is
  a — 0.5 L
  b — 1.5 L
  c — 2.2 L
  d — 4 L
Ans. c

Q55. Most potent stimulus for secretin is
  a — Peristalsis of intestine
  b — Acidic chyme
  c — Protein
  d — Fat
Ans. b

Q56. Which of the following is absorbed in P.C.T
  a — Iron
  b — Electrolytes
  c — Bile salts
  d — V$_1$ + B$_{12}$
Ans. a

Q57. β cells of pancreas produce
  a — Glucagon
  b — Gastrin
  c — Insulin
  d — Pancreatin
Ans. c

Q58. Cell membrane
  a — Consists of protein moleules entirely
  b — Are impermeable to fat soluble substances
  c — In some tissues permit the transport of glucose at the greater rate in presence of insulin
  d — All of the above
Ans. c

Q59. Pancreatic secretion contains
  a — Trypsin
  b — Lipase
  c — Enteropepitidan
  d — Pepsin
  e — Renin
Ans. a, b

Q60. GFR is increased when
  a — Plasma oncotic pressure is increased
  b — Glomerular hydrostatic pressure is decreased
  c — Tubular hydrostatic pressure is increased
  d — Increased renal blood flow
Ans. d

Q61. Chymotrypsinogen is activated to chymotrypsin by
  a — Trypsin
  b — Pepsin
  c — Fatty acids
  d — Bile salts
Ans. a

Multiple choice question

Q62. Most potent bile secreation is
- a — Cholecystokinin
- b — Gastrin
- c — Secretin
- d — Bile gud
- e — Bile salt

Ans. a

Q63. Normal kidney allows passage of
- a — β-globulin
- b — Lysozyme
- c — IgG
- d — Albumin

Ans. a

Q64. Secretin does not cause
- a — Bicarbonate secretion
- b — Augments the action of CCK
- c — Contraction of pyloric sphincter
- d — None of the above

Ans. c

Q65. Somatostatin is produced by
- a — Hypothalamus
- b — Ant. pituitary
- c — Delta cells of pancreas
- d — Alfa cells of pancreas

Ans. c

Q66. SA node is located
- a — Epicardially
- b — Intramyocardial
- c — Subepicardially
- d — Endocardially

Ans. a, c

Q67. Most potent respiratory stimulus is
- a — O_2
- b — CO_2
- c — H^+
- d — K^+

Ans. b

Q68. Melatonin is secreted by
- a — Hypothalamus
- b — Adrenal cortex
- c — Pineal gland
- d — Melanocytes

Ans. c

Q69. Haemophilia is due to deficiency of factor
- a — II
- b — V
- c — VIII
- d — XIII

Ans. c

Q70. Cyanide poisoning effects – functions
- a — Respiratory
- b — Cardial
- c — Renal
- d — Liver

Ans. a

Q71. Rise of pulmonary arterial pressure is caused by
- a — Hypoxia
- b — Acidosis
- c — Alkalosis
- d — All

Ans. a

Q72. Auto regulation is seen in
- a — Liver
- b — Muscle
- c — Kidneys
- d — Brain

Ans. b, c, d

Q73. **Vomiting centre is situated in**
 a — Hypothalamus
 b — Amygdala
 c — Pons
 d — Medulla

Ans. d

Q74. **Medial geniculate body is concerned with**
 a — Hearing
 b — Vision
 c — Smell
 d — Taste

Ans. a

Q75. **Haemophilia is due to deficiency of factor**
 a — II
 b — V
 c — VIII
 d — XIII

Ans. c

Q76. **Cyanide poisoning effects – functions**
 a — Respiratory
 b — Cardial
 c — Renal
 d — Liver

Ans. a

Q77. **Rise of pulmonary arterial pressure is caused by**
 a — Hypoxia
 b — Acidosis
 c — Alkalosis
 d — All

Ans. a

Q78. **Auto regulation is seen in**
 a — Liver
 b — Muscle
 c — Kidneys
 d — Brain

Ans. b, c, d

Q79. **Vomiting centre is situated in**
 a — Hypothalamus
 b — Amygdala
 c — Pons
 d — Medulla

Ans. d

Q80. **Medial geniculate body is concerned with**
 a — Hearing
 b — Vision
 c — Smell
 d — Taste

Ans. a

APPENDIX - I & II

Appendix-I — Investigations with Normal Values

	Males	Females	Units & Method
Hematological Values			
1. Red cell count	4.5 – 6.5	3.8 – 5.8	million / mm^3
2. Haemoglobin	13 – 18	11.5 – 16.5	gm /dl
3. PCV	40 – 54	37 – 47	%
4. ESR (Wintrobes)	0 – 9	0 – 20	mm at end of 1 hour / mm^3
5. TLC	4000 – 11000		
6. DLC	N (40–45), L (20–45), M (2–10), E (1–6), B (<1) %		
7. Platelet count	1.5 – 4 lacs/mm^3		
8. Bleeding time	2 – 7		mins. (Ivy method)
9. Clotting time	3 – 8		mins. (Capillary tube method)
10. Prothrombin time	10 – 16 sec.		
11. Activated partial thromboplastim time	30 – 40 sec.		
12. Thrombin time	10 – 12 sec.		
13. Reticulocyte count	Adults (0.2 – 2%), Infants (2 – 6%)		
Blood Biochemical			
14. Plasma proteins	Total 6.4 – 8.3 gm%, Albumin 3–5 gm%, and Globulin 2 – 3 gm%, A : G ratio – 1.7 : 1		
15. Blood sugar fasting	70 – 90 mg%		
Renal Function Tests			
16. Blood urea	20 – 40 mg%		
17. S. uric acid	3 – 7 mg%		
18. Creatinine	0.7 – 1.5 mg / dl		
19. Creatinine clearance	85 – 130 ml/min		
20. Ketone bodies	0.7 – 1.5 mg%		
21. Urine Albumin	<165 mg / 24 hr.		
Serum Electrolytes			
22. Na$^+$	136 – 145 mEq/l		
23. K$^+$	3.5 – 5 mEq/l		
24. Cl$^-$	96 – 106 mEq/l		
25. HCO$_3$	25 – 50 mEq/l (24-28)		
26. Serum Ca^{++}	9 – 11 mg%		
27. Serum Phosphorous	3 – 4.5 mg%		
Liver Function Tests			
28. Serum bilirubin	Total 0.2 – 1.2 mg/dl; direct 0.1– 0.4 mg%; indirect 0.2 – 0.8 mg%		
29. SGOT (AST)	5 – 40 Units/L (Karmen units)		
30. SGPT (ALT)	5 – 35 Units/L (more specific for liver disease)		
31. Serum alkaline phosphatase	4 – 13 KA units		
Serum Lipids			
32. Serum cholesterol desirable	150 – 240 mg%		
33. LDL cholesterol	<180 mg/dl		
34. VLDL cholesterol	<40 mg/dl		
35. Triglycerides	<165 mg/dl (30–150)		
36. Total lipids	450 – 1000 mg/dl (350 – 800)		
37. FFA	10 – 30 mg%		
Blood Gases			
38. Pressure CO$_2$ (B)	Arteries 40 mmHg; veins 46 mmHg		
O$_2$ (B)	Areries 100 mmHg; veins 40 mmHg		
39. Blood pH	Arterial 7.35 – 7.45 Venous 7.31 – 7.41		
40. Osmolality	289 – 295 mosm / kg of water		

Appendix-II — Some commonly used abbreviations

ACH	Acetylcholine
ADH	Antidiuretic hormone
ATP	Adenosine triphosphate
AV	Atriventricular
BMR	Basal metabolic rate
BP	Blood Pressure
CCK	Cholecystokinin
CNS	Central nerous system
C.O.	Cardiac output
C.S.F.	Cerebrospinal fluid
DNA	Deoxyribonucleic acid
2,3 – DPG	2, 3 – diphosphoglycerate
ECG	Electrocardiogram
EEG	Electroencephalogram
ENS	Enteric nervous system
ESR	Erythrocyte sedmentation rate
FSH	Follicle stimulating hormone
FVC	Forced vital capacity
GFR	Glomerular filtration rate
GH	Growth hormone
GIP	Gastric inhibitory
GnRH	Gonadotropin - Releasing hormone
Hb	Hemoglobin
HbF	Fetal hemoglobin
HbS	Sickle - cell hemoglobin
hCG	Human chorionic gonadotropin
HLA	Human leukocyte antigen
LH	Luteinizing hormone
PTH	Parathyroid hormone
REM	Rapid eye movement
RNA	Ribonucleic acid
T_3	Tri iodothyronine
T_4	Thyroxine
T_m	Transport maximum
TPR	Total peripheral resistance
TSH	Thyroid stimulating hormone
VC	Vital capcity
VIP	Vasoactive intestinal polypeptide

LIST OF FIGURES

Chapter-1: TRANSPORT MECHANISMS
- 1.1 Active process 15
- 1.2 Phagocytosis 16
- 1.3 Pinocytosis 16
- 1.4 Exocytosis 17
- 1.5 Diffusion 17
- 1.6 Dialysis 18
- 1.7 Faciliated diffussion 18

Chapter-2: BODY TISSUES
- 2.1 Skeletal muscle 21
- 2.2 (A) Longitudinal section of skeletal muscle.
  (B) Transverse section of skeletal muscle 22
- 2.3 Mechanism of muscle contraction 23
- 2.4 (A) Longitudinal sections of cardiac muscle.
  (B) Horizontal section of cardiac muscle 24
- 2.5 Cardiac muscle 25
- 2.6 Smooth muscle 25
- 2.7 (A) Lonitudiral section of smooth muscle.
  (B) Horizontal section of smooth muscle 25
- 2.8 A neuron can be unipular, bipolar or multipolar 26
- 2.9 Polarisation an depolarisation in a nerve 28

Chapter-3: BIO-CHEMICAL AND BIO-PHYSICAL PRINCIPLES
- 3.1 Cell with its components 21
- 3.2 Interphase 35
- 3.3 Prophase 36
- 3.4 Metaphase 36
- 3.5 Anaphase 37
- 3.6 Telophase 37
- 3.7 Meiosis 39

Chapter-6: THE BLOOD
- 6.1 Composition of blood 59
- 6.2 The red blood cell 60
- 6.3 The intrinsic and extrinsic pathways of coagulation 69

Chapter-7: THE RETICULOENDOTHELIAL SYSTEM

7.1	The lymphatic system	79
7.2	Diagram showing mechanism of edema	82

Chapter-8: THE CARDIOVASCULAR SYSTEM

8.1	Circulatory system	83
8.2	Composed of circulatory system	84
8.3	Various events in cardiac cycle	86
8.4	The apex beat	88
8.5	Arrangement of different limb leads used to record ECG	89
8.6	Normal electrocardiogram	90
8.7	Distribution of blood volume at rest	91
8.8	Intrinsic autoregulation of cardiac output	94
8.9	The arrangement of the capillary endothelium and astrocyte end-feet in the cerebal circulation	99
8.10	Circulation in skin	101
8.11	The axon reflex	102
8.12	Diagram showing baroreceptors and chemoreceptors	105
8.13	The special conducting system of the heart	108
8.14	Action potential in myocardial cells	109

Chapter-9: THE DIGESTIVE SYSTEM

9.1	The digestive system	113
9.2	Simplified overview of how the energy intake and information occur in body	114
9.3	General plan of different layers in the wall of gut	118
9.4	Secretion of saliva	120
9.5	Structure involved in swollowing	121
9.6	Parts of stomach	122
9.7	Factors influencing gastrin secretion	123
9.8	Mechanism of secretion of gastric paid	124
9.9	Small intestine	126
9.10	Peristaltic movements in small intestine	127
9.11	The large intestine	128
9.12	Defecation reflex	129
9.13	Entrohepatic circulation of bile salts	130
9.14	Glucose absorption from intestinal site	133
9.15	Summary of digestion and obsorption of lipids	134

9.16 Absorption of amino acids 135
9.17 Biological value of some common food proteins 136

Chapter-10: THE INTEGUMENTARY SYSTEM
10.1 Skin and hair 137

Chapter-11: THE RESPIRATORY SYSTEM
11.1   Respiratory system 143
11.2   Trachea and lungs 144
11.3   Respiratory membrane 146
11.4   Lung showing the pleura 146
11.5   The respiratory unit 147
11.6   Respiratory movements 148
11.7   Pulmonary volumes and capacities 150
11.8   Compliance diagram of lung 151
11.9   Surfactant 152
11.10 Gas diffusion 154
11.11 Oxygen transport 156
11.12 The haemoglobin dissociation curve 156
11.13 Summary of CO_2 transport in the blood 158
11.14 Equilibration of blood and tissue gases 160

Chapter-12: THE EXCRETORY SYSTEM
12.1   Kidney 165
12.2   (A) The excretory system.
       (B) Structure of kidney in detail 166
12.3   Nephron 167
12.4   Juxta glomerular apparatus 172
12.5   Reabsorption of amino acids in proximal tubles 173
12.6   Bicarbonate reabsorption in proximal tubule 173
12.7   Secretion of organic anions into lumen
       of proximal tubule 174
12.8   Uptake of Na^+ and Cl^- in thick ascending
       limb of loop of henle 175
12.9   Secretion of potassium ions in distal
       tubule and collecting duct 175

Chapter-13: THE NERVOUS SYSTEM
13.1   Nervous system 179
13.2   Transverse section of spinal cord showing
       arrangement of white and grey matter 181

13.3 Types of synapses :
    (a) Axo-somatic.
    (b) Axo-dendritic.
    (c) Dentro-dentritic.
    (d) Axo-axonal 184
13.4 Basic neuronal circuit of stretch reflex 186
13.5 Somatotrophic organization of different body parts in somatosensory cortex 188
13.6 Respresertation of body in motor cortex 190
13.7 Pyramidal pathways 191
13.8 The autonomic nervous system 193
13.9 The vestibular apparatus 195
13.10 Structure of crista 196
13.11 Neural pathways from vestibular apparatus 197
13.12 Response of hair cells when a semicircular canal is rotated and then stoped 197
13.13 The basal ganglia 200
13.14 Connections of basal ganglia 201
13.15 With increasing age there is decrease in the hours of sleep and also the portion of REM sleep decreases with age 203
13.16 The fundamental neural organization of the cerebellar 205
13.17 Layer of cerebellar cortex 206
13.18 Cerebruspinal fluid pathway. The black arrow show the pathway of cerebrospinal fluid flow from choroid in the lateral ventricles to the arachnoid villi 206

Chapter-14: THE SENSE ORGANS

14.1 Eye and ears 209
14.2 Structure of eye 210
14.3 Structure of lens 212
14.4 Gross anatomy of theretria 212
14.5 Microscopic structure of retina 213
14.6 Emmetropic eye 215
14.7 Hypermetropic eye 216
14.8 Correction of hypermetropic eye using a conves lens ..216
14.9 Refraction of myopic eye 216
14.10 Correction of myopic eye using a concave lens 217
14.11 The visual pathways. Damage to the stracts at the location indicates causes defects in the visual fields as shown in the diagram on the right 218

14.12 Dark adaptation 219
14.13 Various extraocular muscles producing
 movements of the eyeball 220
14.14 Accommodation at rest 221
14.15 Accommotion 221
14.16 Taste sensation 222
14.17 Neural pathway 222
14.18 General senstion (other than taste) 223
14.19 Olfactory apparatus 223
14.20 The olfactory pathway 224
14.21 Components of the ear 225
14.22 Section through cochlea showing the three
 compartments
 R — Reissuer's membrane
 B — Basilar membrane
 C — Tectorical membrane 226
14.23 The laryngeal framework 228
14.24 A diagram of the left hemisphere to show the
 location of the principal region involved in the control
 of speech, 1 & 2 indicate the postulated connection
 between the primary visiual and auditory receiving
 area, and the language area of the temporal lobe
 and angular gyrus. 3 indicates the connection
 between the angular gyrus and broca's area via
 the arcuate fasciculus 229

Chapter-15: ENDOCRINE SYSTEM
 15.1 Hormone secreting glands and cells 231

Chapter-16: REPRODUCTION
 16.1 Male reproductive system 248
 16.2 Spermatogensis 249
 16.3 Section of testis showing stages of spermatogensis 249
 16.4 Female reporductive system 252
 16.5 The female gential tract 253
 16.6 Oogenesis 254
 16.7 The menstrual cycle 255
 16.8 Hormonal interactions in the ovarion
  and uterine cycles 257
 16.9 The female breast 258